STUDY GUIDE FOR ADVANCED LIFE SUPPORT
PROBLEM SOLVING IN CARDIAC ARREST

STUDY GUIDE FOR ADVANCED LIFE SUPPORT

PROBLEM SOLVING IN CARDIAC ARREST

KEN GRAUER, M.D., F.A.A.F.P.

ACLS Affiliate Faculty, Assistant Professor,
Department of Community Health and Family Medicine,
University of Florida, College of Medicine,
Gainesville, Florida

With **232** *illustrations*

The C. V. Mosby Company

ST. LOUIS • TORONTO • PRINCETON   1984

MOSBY

A TRADITION OF PUBLISHING EXCELLENCE

Editor: Carol Trumbold
Assistant editor: Anne Gunter
Manuscript editor: Selena V. Bussen
Book design: Staff
Production: Jeanne A. Gulledge

The C.V. Mosby Company
11830 Westline Industrial Drive, St. Louis, Missouri 63146

Library of Congress Cataloging in Publication Data

Grauer, Ken.
  Study guide for advanced life support.

  Bibliography: p.
  Includes index.
  1. Cardiac arrest—Treatment—Problems, exercises, etc.
2. Cardiac resuscitation—Problems, exercises, etc.
I. Title. [DNLM: 1. Heart arrest—Therapy—Handbooks.
2. Resuscitation—Handbooks. WG 205 G774s]
RC685.C173G73   1984   616.1'206   83-19517
ISBN 0-8016-1878-9

TS/VH/VH   9 8 7 6 5 4 3 2 1   03/D/327

To Michelle
   for her patience and love

Foreword

Advanced cardiac life support (ACLS) is a program designed by the American Heart Association for teaching health care professionals a systematic approach to the treatment of cardiac arrest and other acute cardiac-related problems. The success of this program nationally has become evident from the increasing demand for ACLS training, with approximately 25,000 health care professionals taught in 1982.

The participant of an ACLS course is expected to assimilate a tremendous amount of material. In our institution we have recognized the difficulty of trying to teach this material in the short 2- to 3-day period that is usually allotted for the course. Even though the American Heart Association ACLS textbook is distributed well in advance, it has not solved the problem of preparing the student for the intensive course to follow. Although comprehensive, the ACLS textbook does not organize material into a decision-making format for patient care.

Study Guide for Advanced Life Support: Problem Solving in Cardiac Arrest has been developed in an attempt to meet this need. The reader becomes actively involved in the decision-making process by working through case studies in cardiac arrest that closely simulate the content of the ACLS skill stations of defibrillation, dysrhythmia recognition, and MEGA CODE. Additional didactic sections thoroughly review pharmacologic principles and offer more practice in dysrhythmia interpretation. Numerous tables and a series of algorithms summarize

the management of cardiac arrest. The style of the book is easy to read yet informative, and the interest of those with either a limited or advanced medical background is sustained throughout.

The rapidly changing field of emergency cardiac care has made it difficult to delineate specific guidelines for managing cardiac arrest. Grauer has met this challenge head on. He discusses standard treatment protocols yet also explores new innovative developments in management that have been suggested since the ACLS textbook was published.

We feel that *Study Guide for Advanced Life Support* will be of value to anyone taking the ACLS course and will serve as an extremely useful reference for those involved in emergency cardiac care. We find it both stimulating and informative.

RICHARD J. MELKER, M.D., Ph.D.
National ACLS Affiliate Faculty,
Assistant Professor,
Surgery, Anesthesiology, Pediatrics,
University of Florida,
College of Medicine,
Gainesville, Florida

DANIEL L. CAVALLARO, REMT
Assistant in Surgery,
Director, Advanced Life Support Training,
University of Florida,
College of Medicine,
Gainesville, Florida

Preface

The outlook for victims of cardiac arrest has improved greatly during the past decade. Thanks to community programs on cardiopulmonary resuscitation (CPR), a more informed public is better able to recognize cardiac arrest and initiate basic life support (BLS), and more widespread emergency medical systems (EMS) capable of providing advanced life support (ALS) are reaching victims sooner. Over 50% of people who are not in a hospital and experience cardiac arrest are now successfully resuscitated in communities like Seattle with ultimate discharge home in about half of these cases. This almost doubles success rates prevalent during the early 1970s. The prognosis of patients who experience cardiac arrest within the hospital has also improved, principally, as the result of the increased familiarity of hospital staff with the techniques of resuscitation. Perhaps in no other area of medicine has the command of a body of knowledge and its instant application been so important in determining survival.

The skills and concepts of cardiac resuscitation have been refined and synthesized into a core of practical knowledge by the National Conference on Cardiopulmonary Resuscitation and Emergency Cardiac Care. Its guidelines are taught in advanced cardiac life support (ACLS) courses that have trained thousands of physicians, nurses, medical students, paramedics, and other paramedical personnel across the country. What about the professional who is not well versed in these techniques either because of inadequate previous exposure to acutely ill patients or a primary interest in other fields of medicine? The confidence and ability to make split second decisions on diagnosis and treatment of life-threatening dysrhythmias may be lacking when the need arises if it has not been sufficiently practiced beforehand.

The purpose of this text is to review the essentials of managing cardiac arrest. Diagnosis of the various dysrhythmias encountered during a code situation is stressed along with a rationale for appropriate therapy. The book is unique in its approach. It does not follow the more conventional plan of classifying dysrhythmias according to their site of origin (atrial, atrioventricular [AV] nodal, or ventricular dysrhythmias) and separating their diagnosis from treatment. Instead it examines the natural sequence of events that occur during a cardiac arrest and integrates a practical approach to both diagnosis and therapeutic decision making.

The book has been written for the noncardiologist. It is equally pertinent to all medical personnel who participate in cardiac resuscitation, regardless of their prior level of training. It does not attempt to supplant the guidelines put forth by the 1979 National Conference on Cardiopulmonary Resuscitation and Emergency Cardiac Care but rather reinforces them in a way that challenges the reader and allows application of knowledge.

I am indebted to the following people whose contributions were instrumental to the preparation of this book:

R. Whitney Curry, Jr., M.D., Associate Professor, Director Family Practice Residency Program, University of Florida, Gainesville; and Daniel L. Cavallaro, REMT, Advanced Life Support Program Director, College of Medicine, University of Florida, Gainesville, for their expertise in reviewing the majority of the text.

Holly Jensen, R.N., and Michelle C. Grauer, R.N., CCRN for supplying part of the electrocardiograms.

J. Daniel Robinson, Pharm.D. for contributing the SIMKIN figures on lidocaine.

Paul Arons, M.D.; William Goellner, M.D.; Michelle C. Grauer, R.N., CCRN; Ralph Guild, M.D.; Eloise Harman, M.D.; Holly Jensen, R.N.; Tom Kemp; Jack Kravitz, M.D.; Larry Kravitz, M.D.; Jim Nimocks, M.D.; James R. Piotrowski, P.A.; J. Daniel Robinson, Pharm.D.; Glenn Siegfried, M.D.; Kay Staniszewski, R.N., CCRN; Maura Sughrue, M.D.; and Eileen Weimerskirch, M.D. for the constructive commentary offered on selected portions of the text.

All the cardiologists from whom I have learned.

KEN GRAUER

How to use this book

This book has been functionally divided into four parts to suit the needs of the reader. Part I offers a brief overview of cardiopulmonary resuscitation. It includes six algorithms that summarize a suggested treatment protocol for cardiac arrest, a section on pitfalls in current techniques and new trends in management, and a drug compendium of the most commonly used pharmacologic agents in emergency cardiac care.

The algorithms provide an overall perspective of the management of cardiac arrest. They may be used either as a study guide while the reader is working through the clinical case studies or as a ready review for quick referral. Although one may object to the use of algorithms because they sometimes restrict thinking and do not always apply to the particular situation, their use in the management of cardiac arrest has been shown to expedite clinical decision making. In an emergency situation such as cardiopulmonary arrest, the ability to rapidly decide on an effective course of therapy is probably the most important factor affecting survival. Algorithms supply the basic framework from which the emergency care provider can expediently organize thinking, set priorities, and initiate an appropriate therapeutic approach. They do not account for all of the possible permutations of management; to do so would require specification of an endless number of uncommonly used alternatives that would only confuse the issue and defeat the original purpose of the algorithm.

The section on pitfalls in current techniques and new trends in management enumerates a number of errors commonly committed during cardiopulmonary resuscitation. Delivery of emergency cardiac care may improve with increased awareness of these factors. Attention is drawn to oversights such as not using the quick-look paddles, not applying 25 pounds of firm pressure to each paddle when defibrillating, and forgetting about the intratracheal route for drug administration. Also included in this section is a list of indications for emergency cardiac pacing, a short discussion on the detection and management of electromechanical dissociation and on new developments in CPR, and a list of pitfalls in dysrhythmia interpretation. Finally, the section on new trends in the pharmacologic management of cardiac arrest reviews a number of important concepts about the use of nine essential drugs in cardiac resuscitation. Suggestions are made in the current treatment protocol incorporating these concepts with recent developments in the field.

The drug compendium features an easy reference table that summarizes the actions, indications, doses, and adverse effects of the most frequently used drugs in emergency cardiac care. A separate table of drug doses in pediatric resuscitation follows. Calculation of intravenous infusion rates is thoroughly explained, and a method for remembering how to set up intravenous infusions is presented. A special discussion on the use of lidocaine addresses why so many protocols exist for the administration of this commonly used antiarrhythmic agent. Understanding the pharmacokinetics of the drug allows one to optimize drug delivery and minimize the risk of toxicity.

Part II presents a systematic approach to dysrhythmia interpretation. Specific problems that commonly confront the emergency care provider (diagnosing tachydysrhythmias, differentiating premature ventricular contractions [PVCs] from aberrancy, and determining the degree of heart block) are covered in an easy-to-follow informative style that actively recruits participation of the reader. Clinical relevancy is stressed.

Principles discussed in these first two parts are applied in the case studies that constitute Part III. The reader is transported to the scene of a patient with cardiac arrest (either at the bedside or in the field) and asked to assume direction of the resuscitative efforts. Greatest benefit may be derived by actively working through these case studies in the order in which they are presented and referring back to material covered in Parts I and II as needed. Alternatively,

one may choose to begin the book with these case studies and selectively refer to the algorithms, drug compendium, or dysrhythmia section as questions arise.

The reader may assess general knowledge on cardiac resuscitation in Part IV. Fifty multiple choice and true or false questions make up the first portion of this part and test the general knowledge of the subject. By checking answers with those provided and using the referenced pages in the American Heart Association's (AHA) *Textbook of Advanced Cardiac Life Support* and/or the *JAMA Supplement* when needed, the reader may use this test as an aid in preparing for the written portion of a formal course in advanced life support.

The 50 rhythm strips in the second portion of Part IV offer a final challenge to the reader. Detailed answers explain the rationale for arriving at each interpretation and review many of the concepts covered in the book. Scoring well in this portion should correlate with proficiency in recognizing dysrhythmias encountered in emergency cardiac care.

Contents

PART ONE

OVERVIEW OF CARDIOPULMONARY RESUSCITATION

CHAPTER 1

Algorithms for treatment

This chapter provides a brief overview of the approach to the victim of cardiopulmonary arrest and introduces the algorithms for treatment. Most cases of cardiopulmonary arrest occur outside the hospital. The key to survival lies with early recognition of the clinical state of unresponsiveness (apnea or pulselessness), initiation of basic life support by the lay public, and activation of emergency medical system (EMS) personnel.

Assessment and management of the unconscious victim begin with the ABCs of cardiopulmonary resuscitation. Once unresponsiveness has been established and help has been called, the rescuer should open the airway and check for the existence and adequacy of spontaneous breathing and circulation. If the patient is not breathing, mouth-to-mouth ventilation should be attempted. This results in expansion of the chest if the airway is patent. With airway obstruction the chest does not rise; maneuvers to relieve airway obstruction (repositioning the patient, applying back blows, manual thrusts, and the finger sweep) take precedence over further attempts at ventilation.

Once a patent airway has been established, four full breaths are delivered. The status of the circulation is next assessed. If no carotid pulse is palpable, external chest compression must be started immediately.

The combination of external chest compression and artificial ventilation constitutes the *basic life support* measures of cardiopulmonary resuscitation. They may be accomplished by one or preferably two individuals and should be continued by the initial rescuer(s) until effective spontaneous circulation and ventilation have been restored, resuscitative efforts have been transferred to better trained personnel, or the rescuer is exhausted and is unable to continue with the resuscitation.

Once providers capable of administering advanced life support arrive, attention may be directed to delivery of more definitive therapy. The choice of treatment depends on the precipitating (primary) mechanism of the arrest. If the patient is found in *ventricular fibrillation*, immediate defibrillation is indicated. The chance of survival is inversely related to the amount of time from the onset of ventricular fibrillation until countershock is applied. *Ventricular tachycardia* with hemodynamic compromise also requires immediate electrical conversion. On the other hand, patients with *bradydysrhythmias* (including asystole and electromechanical dissociation) are first treated medically (with epinephrine, sodium bicarbonate, etc). These three dysrhythmias make up the principle primary mechanisms of cardiopulmonary arrest (upper panel of Algorithm A). Suggested protocols for management are outlined in Algorithms B, C, and D.

Text continued on p. 10.

3

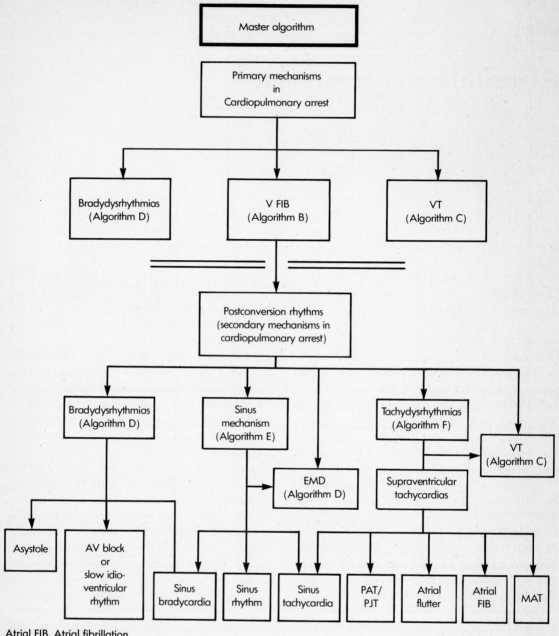

Atrial FIB, Atrial fibrillation
EMD, Electromechanical dissociation
MAT, Multifocal atrial tachycardia
PAT, Paroxysmal atrial tachycardia
PJT, Paroxysmal junctional tachycardia
V FIB, Ventricular fibrillation
VT, Ventricular tachycardia

Algorithm A

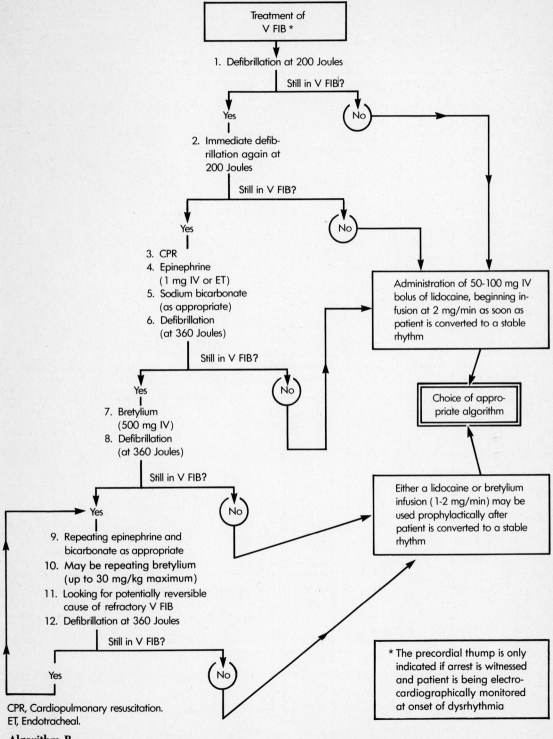

Treatment of V FIB *

1. Defibrillation at 200 Joules

Still in V FIB?

Yes — No

2. Immediate defibrillation again at 200 Joules

Still in V FIB?

Yes — No

3. CPR
4. Epinephrine (1 mg IV or ET)
5. Sodium bicarbonate (as appropriate)
6. Defibrillation (at 360 Joules)

Still in V FIB?

Yes — No

Administration of 50-100 mg IV bolus of lidocaine, beginning infusion at 2 mg/min as soon as patient is converted to a stable rhythm

7. Bretylium (500 mg IV)
8. Defibrillation (at 360 Joules)

Still in V FIB?

Yes — No

Choice of appropriate algorithm

9. Repeating epinephrine and bicarbonate as appropriate
10. May be repeating bretylium (up to 30 mg/kg maximum)
11. Looking for potentially reversible cause of refractory V FIB
12. Defibrillation at 360 Joules

Still in V FIB?

Yes — No

Either a lidocaine or bretylium infusion (1-2 mg/min) may be used prophylactically after patient is converted to a stable rhythm

* The precordial thump is only indicated if arrest is witnessed and patient is being electrocardiographically monitored at onset of dysrhythmia

CPR, Cardiopulmonary resuscitation.
ET, Endotracheal.

Algorithm B

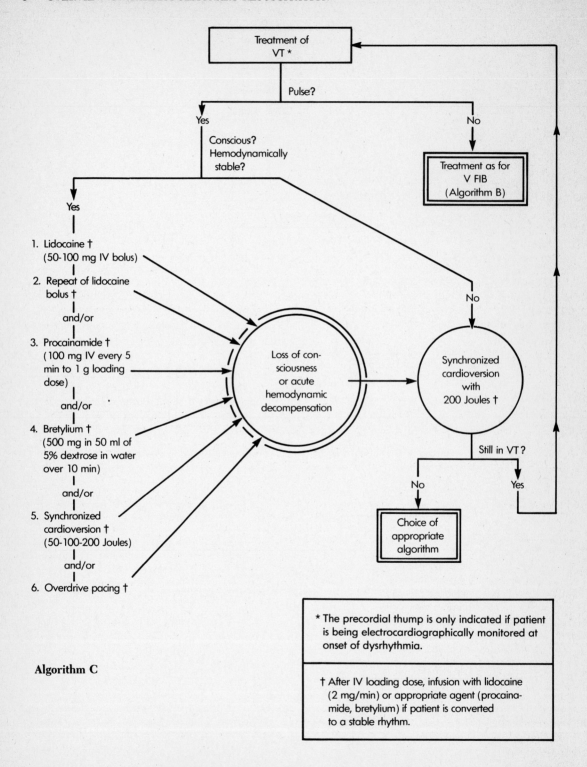

Treatment of VT *

Pulse?

Yes — Conscious? Hemodynamically stable?

No — Treatment as for V FIB (Algorithm B)

Yes:

1. Lidocaine † (50-100 mg IV bolus)
2. Repeat of lidocaine bolus †

   and/or

3. Procainamide † (100 mg IV every 5 min to 1 g loading dose)

   and/or

4. Bretylium † (500 mg in 50 ml of 5% dextrose in water over 10 min)

   and/or

5. Synchronized cardioversion † (50-100-200 Joules)

   and/or

6. Overdrive pacing †

No → Loss of consciousness or acute hemodynamic decompensation → Synchronized cardioversion with 200 Joules †

Still in VT?

No → Choice of appropriate algorithm

Yes

Algorithm C

* The precordial thump is only indicated if patient is being electrocardiographically monitored at onset of dysrhythmia.

† After IV loading dose, infusion with lidocaine (2 mg/min) or appropriate agent (procainamide, bretylium) if patient is converted to a stable rhythm.

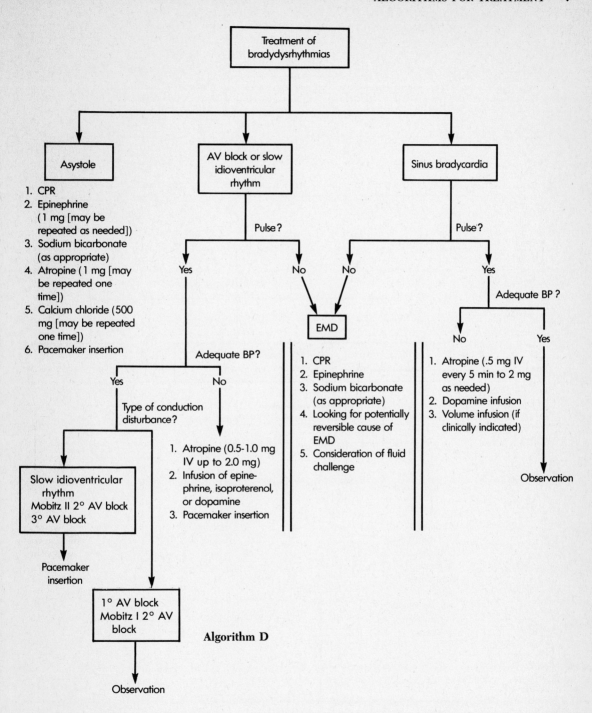

Algorithm D

BP, Blood pressure.

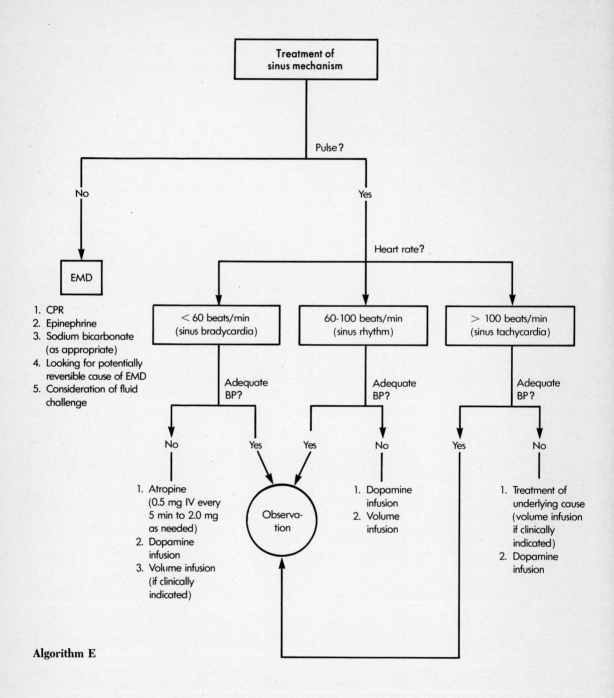

Algorithm E

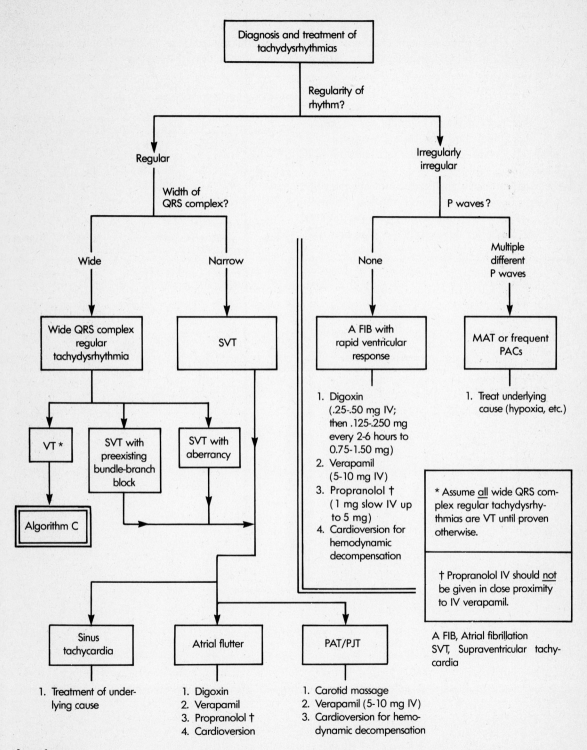

Diagnosis and treatment of tachydysrhythmias

Regularity of rhythm?

Regular

Irregularly irregular

Width of QRS complex?

P waves?

Wide

Narrow

None

Multiple different P waves

Wide QRS complex regular tachydysrhythmia

SVT

A FIB with rapid ventricular response

MAT or frequent PACs

VT *

SVT with preexisting bundle-branch block

SVT with aberrancy

Algorithm C

1. Digoxin (.25-.50 mg IV; then .125-.250 mg every 2-6 hours to 0.75-1.50 mg)
2. Verapamil (5-10 mg IV)
3. Propranolol † (1 mg slow IV up to 5 mg)
4. Cardioversion for hemodynamic decompensation

1. Treat underlying cause (hypoxia, etc.)

* Assume all wide QRS complex regular tachydysrhythmias are VT until proven otherwise.

† Propranolol IV should not be given in close proximity to IV verapamil.

Sinus tachycardia

Atrial flutter

PAT/PJT

A FIB, Atrial fibrillation
SVT, Supraventricular tachycardia

1. Treatment of underlying cause

1. Digoxin
2. Verapamil
3. Propranolol †
4. Cardioversion

1. Carotid massage
2. Verapamil (5-10 mg IV)
3. Cardioversion for hemodynamic decompensation

Algorithm F

The lower panel in Algorithm A indicates the possible secondary mechanisms that may develop during cardiopulmonary arrest if the patient is converted out of ventricular fibrillation. In addition to ventricular tachycardia and brady-dysrhythmias, ventricular fibrillation may be converted to a *sinus mechanism* or *tachydys-rhythmia*. Suggested treatment protocols for these latter two possibilities are outlined in Algorithms E and F.

Although these algorithms could not possibly encompass every conceivable clinical situation that might arise during cardiopulmonary resuscitation, they offer the emergency care provider a concise yet practical plan for therapeutic decision making in the management of cardiac arrest and outline the treatment strategy employed in this text.

SUGGESTED READINGS

American Heart Association Subcommittee on Emergency Cardiac Care: Standards and guidelines for cardiopulmonary resuscitation (CPR) and emergency cardiac care (ECC), JAMA **244**:453-509, 1980.

Auerbach, P.S., and Budassi, S.A., (editors): Cardiac arrest and CPR, Rockville, Md., 1983, Aspen Systems Corp.

McIntyre, K.M., and Lewis, J.A., (editors): Textbook of advanced cardiac life support, Dallas, 1981, American Heart Association.

Safar, P.: Cardiopulmonary cerebral resuscitation, Stavanger, Norway, 1981, Asmund S. Laerdal.

CHAPTER 2

Pitfalls in current techniques and new trends in management

The techniques of basic and advanced cardiac life support have been taught to thousands of medical and paramedical personnel across the country. Yet despite this widespread dispersion of knowledge, certain fundamental mistakes in the application of these techniques continue to occur on a frequent basis. In addition, the past few years have seen a number of new developments in the management of cardiac arrest, especially in regard to pharmacologic therapy. The purpose of this section is to review some of the pitfalls in our current techniques of cardiopulmonary resuscitation and discuss some of the newer trends in management ideally so that this information will be useful in improving the delivery of emergency cardiac care.

GENERAL MANAGEMENT OF CARDIAC ARREST

Listed below are common problems encountered in the general management of cardiac arrest.

1. *Failure of someone to assume command of directing the code.* This does not necessarily have to be a physician but may be the first qualified emergency care provider on the scene. Whether this role is subsequently passed on to more knowledgeable authorities as they arrive is not nearly as important as having a single person clearly defined as the one responsible for making decisions.

Some of the many roles of the *code director* are to

a. Oversee and coordinate the overall resuscitative effort.

b. Clear the room of unnecessary personnel.

c. Verify that CPR is being done correctly and that a pulse is produced by external chest compressions.

d. Make sure that breath sounds are checked following endotracheal intubation.

e. Make sure that a pulse is checked for whenever the cardiac rhythm changes. If a pulse is present, a blood pressure must be checked.

f. Order the administration of drugs in the appropriate dosage and by the appropriate route.

g. Delegate a specific individual to inquire about the patient's history, his overall health status, and the events leading up to the arrest. Resuscitation of a person with diabetes in ketoacidosis is vastly different from resuscitation of a patient who has overdosed or is

11

exsanguinating. Moreover, how aggressively one proceeds with the resuscitative effort may be strongly influenced by factors in the patient's history, such as whether or not he has a terminal disease.

h. Order appropriate radiographic and laboratory tests as they are needed. Arterial blood gases (ABGs) should be drawn as soon as possible to guide therapy with sodium bicarbonate. Once a stable rhythm is established, a chest x-ray film should be done to verify correct positioning of the endotracheal tube, central lines, and/or pacemaker wires and to rule out pneumothorax. Finally, serum electrolyte concentrations and other blood work may be needed to assist in determining the etiology of the arrest.

i. Consult with the patient's primary physician at the earliest opportunity.

j. Talk to the paient's family.

k. Decide when the resuscitation effort should be terminated.

2. *Failure to record the sequence of events as they unfold during the arrest.*
The *code sheet* should reflect the following information:

a. The various cardiac rhythms that occurred during the code and whether or not they were associated with a pulse and blood pressure.

b. The time of administration, dose, and indication for all medications given during the code.

c. The number of countershock attempts and the energies used.

d. The performance of any procedures such as endotracheal intubation, pericardiocentesis, or insertion of a pacemaker or of central IV lines.

e. The names of the emergency care providers in attendance.

f. The time the arrest began and the time and reason the resuscitation effort was terminated.

Keeping track of this information during the code is particularly important with regard to the administration of drugs such as sodium bicarbonate. Correlation of the time of administration with respect to the timing of endotracheal intubation and of drawing the ABGs is critical. Medicolegally, the code sheet provides documentation. It is extremely difficult to reconstruct the sequence of events after the code.

3. *Not regularly checking to see that all crash cart drugs are restocked and all emergency equipment is in working order.* Laryngoscope bulbs, Ambu bags, and suction equipment tend to be missing at the moment they are needed for a call of cardiac arrest. Similarly, essential drugs such as epinephrine, dopamine, and bretylium may not be available when needed unless provisions for regularly scheduled crash cart maintenance checks have been made.

4. *Failure to consider "Do Not Resuscitate" (DNR) orders* before *the cardiac arrest occurs.* A routine practice should be made when admitting any patient to the hospital of assessing whether or not resuscitation efforts should be initiated in the event of a cardiopulmonary arrest. This decision should be arrived at jointly by the physicians caring for the patient, the patient's family, and the patient himself if he is competent to participate in the decision-making process. If the patient's condition subsequently changes during the course of hospitalization, the decision regarding whether or not to initiate resuscitation may need to be reconsidered. If it is felt to be in the patient's best interests not to initiate cardiopulmonary resuscitation (CPR) because of a terminal illness, etc., this decision must be adequately documented on the chart and made clear to all hospital personnel involved in the care of the patient.

PROVISION OF BASIC AND ADVANCED LIFE SUPPORT

Listed below are common problems encountered in providing basic and advanced life support.

1. *Delay in making the diagnosis of cardiopulmonary arrest.* As soon as unresponsiveness has been verified, it is imperative to call for help while checking for the adequacy of spontaneous ventilation and circulation. Basic life support must be started promptly for pulselessness and/or apnea.

2. *Delay in securing an airway.* The resuscitation is doomed to failure unless an airway can be established and maintained. CPR should not be repeatedly interrupted by inexpert attempts at intubation, since ventilation with a properly positioned mask usually is sufficient to maintain adequate oxygenation until personnel experienced in intubation arrive.

3. *Failure to place a bed board under the patient.* Cardiac massage is not effective when performed on a mattress.

4. *Unnecessarily interrupting CPR.* CPR should not be stopped for more than 5 seconds except for intubating or moving the patient. No more than 30 seconds interruption is permitted for these maneuvers.

5. *Improper application of external chest compression.* The rescuer should be correctly positioned over the patient's sternum with arms extended while pressure is applied to the lower sternum with the heels of both hands. The sternum should be displaced by 1½ to 2 inches toward the spine. The rescuer should not remove his or her hands from the sternum between compressions but must release pressure completely. Fingers should not rest on the patient's chest, and jerking or bouncing movements must be avoided. Instead, external chest compression should be smooth and regular and occupy at least 50% of the cycle to assure maximum blood flow during CPR.*

6. *Misuse of the precordial thump.* Although the precordial thump may restore sinus rhythm if delivered soon after the onset of ventricular tachycardia or ventricular fibrillation, it may occasionally cause asystole. As a result, the precordial thump should no longer be routinely applied at the onset of CPR. The only circumstance for which the precordial thump is now recommended is when an emergency care provider personally observes the onset of ventricular tachycardia or ventricular fibrillation in a patient who is already being electrocardiographically monitored.

7. *Ignoring gastric distention.* Even when performed correctly, CPR may result in gastric distention. This can compromise left ventricular filling and predispose the patient to regurgitation of stomach contents. Increasing gastric distention during CPR should be recognized and relieved by early insertion of a nasogastric tube after protecting the airway by endotracheal intubation.

8. *Unnecessary concern with sterile techniques during resuscitation.*

9. *Preoccupation with inserting a central line.* During closed chest compression, circulation of drugs by a central IV line is preferable to using a peripheral IV (Kuhn et al., 1981). Use of a central IV allows immediate access into the central circulation and accommodates a larger volume than a peripheral IV. However, insertion of an internal jugular or subclavian line requires cessation of CPR and exposes the patient to a significant risk of pneumothorax. Though these disadvantages

---

*At the time of this writing, the mechanism by which blood is circulated during external chest compressions is under reinvestigation. (See section on new developments in CPR.)

do not apply to the insertion of a femoral line, blood flow during CPR may be diminished below the diaphragm (Dalsey et al., 1983; Niemann et al., 1981), perhaps making this central IV route less desirable. Since circulation of drugs administered by a peripheral IV is usually sufficient to allow adequate blood flow during cardiac resuscitation, early insertion of a central line should probably be avoided unless the physician is highly skilled in this technique.

10. *Forgetting about the intratracheal route.* The onset of action of intratracheally administered epinephrine in patients with cardiovascular collapse is comparable to the drug given intravenously (Parmley et al., 1982; Redding, 1979). Thus in the event that a patient is intubated but an IV line cannot be started, one should not hesitate to give epinephrine through the endotracheal tube. Atropine and lidocaine may also be administered by this route. (The mnemonic *A L E* [*a*tropine, *l*idocaine, *e*pinephrine] may help to recall these three drugs.)

11. *Failure to flush the IV line after the administration of sodium bicarbonate.* Catecholamines (epinephrine, dopamine, isoproterenol) and calcium salts are inactivated when mixed with sodium bicarbonate. For this reason the IV line must be flushed after giving sodium bicarbonate before infusing additional drugs. From a practical standpoint it would therefore seem preferable to administer epinephrine *before* giving sodium bicarbonate. A smaller volume of epinephine (1 mg ampule is 10 ml) can be given much more rapidly than a larger volume of sodium bicarbonate (50 mEq ampule is 50 ml), and one does not have to flush the IV line after the epinephrine has been given. (Alternatively, if both an endotracheal tube and IV line are in place, one might optimize drug delivery by the simultaneous administration of epinephrine down the endotracheal tube with the peripheral infusion of sodium bicarbonate.)

12. *Inappropriate administration of medication by intracardiac injection.* This route of drug administration should be reserved as a last resort because of the unjustifiably high incidence of complications associated with its use. These include induction of intractable ventricular fibrillation, laceration of a coronary artery, pneumothorax, and hemopericardium with tamponade.

13. *Forgetting that atropine administration is a common cause of dilated pupils during cardiac arrest.* The resuscitation effort should not be terminated because of pupillary unresponsiveness if atropine was administered during the code.

14. *Failure to actively seek out an underlying cause of electromechanical dissociation (EMD).* (See section on detection and management of EMD.)

15. *Delay in arranging for emergency pacing.* A patient with a hemodynamically significant bradydysrhythmia who has not responded to atropine is in need of cardiac pacing. The use of agents such as isoproterenol should *only* be employed as a stopgap measure to support the patient until the pacemaker has been inserted. (See section on indications for emergency cardiac pacing.)

DEFIBRILLATION

Listed below are common problems encountered when defibrillating a patient.

1. *Forgetting to clear the area before defibrillation.* Although this may seem obvious, the careless application of countershock without first verifying that no one is in direct or indirect contact with the patient still results in accidental defibrillations of hospital personnel.

2. *Failure to apply 25 pounds of firm arm*

pressure to each paddle when defibrillating. Application of firm pressure to the chest wall reduces transthoracic resistance and increases the efficacy of defibrillation.

3. *Unfamiliarity with the defibrillation equipment*.

4. *Failure to use the quick-look paddles*. Most defibrillators are equipped to provide a quick look at the cardiac rhythm on contact of the paddles to the patient's chest. This saves the time of applying monitoring leads, and in the case of ventricular fibrillation it allows for more rapid initial defibrillation.

5. *Delay in defibrillation*. The chance of successful conversion of ventricular fibrillation is inversely proportional to the time from the onset of this rhythm until countershock is applied. Thus one should defibrillate the patient immediately after confirming the diagnosis of ventricular fibrillation rather than losing time trying to first intubate or secure an IV line.

6. *Use of excessive energy with initial defibrillation attempts*. Weaver et al. (1982) have shown that initial defibrillation with 175 J of delivered energy is as effective in converting ventricular fibrillation as countershock with 320 J, yet it is associated with a lower incidence of advanced atrioventricular (AV) block after defibrillation. Consequently, the delivered energy of the initial two countershock attempts should probably be limited to 200 J. If this is unsuccessful, subsequent attempts at defibrillation should be with 300 to 360 J.

7. *Forgetting to immediately deliver a second countershock if the initial attempt at defibrillation is unsuccessful*. Successive countershocks reduce transthoracic resistance, making the second attempt more effective.

8. *Failure to use synchronized cardioversion when indicated*. Synchronized cardiover-

sion is indicated for the treatment of patients with supraventricular tachycardias or ventricular tachycardia if they demonstrate hemodynamic compromise. By delivering the electrical impulse during that portion of the cardiac cycle when the ventricles are most refractory, synchronized cardioversion is less likely to cause ventricular fibrillation than unsynchronized countershock.

9. *Forgetting to administer lidocaine prophylactically following successful conversion of ventricular fibrillation*.

DYSRHYTHMIA INTERPRETATION

Listed below are common problems encountered in interpreting dysrhythmias.

1. *Forgetting that the most common reason for a pause is a blocked premature atrial contraction (PAC) and not heart block*.

2. *Not distinguishing between AV dissociation and complete AV block*.

3. *Misdiagnosing second-degree AV block with 2:1 AV conduction as Mobitz II*.

4. *Failure to recognize and appreciate the diagnostic use of group beating* (often implies a Wenckebach-type block).

5. *Misdiagnosis of accelerated idioventricular rhythm (AIVR) as ventricular tachycardia* (and mistreating the dysrhythmia with lidocaine or countershock).

6. *Falsely assuming a wide complex tachydysrhythmia is supraventricular because the patient is alert and hemodynamically stable*.

7. *Not suspecting atrial flutter with a supraventricular tachycardia that has a ventricular response of about 150 beats/min*.

8. *Not recognizing atrial fibrillation when the ventricular response is rapid and only a minor degree of irregularity exists*.

9. *Falsely assuming anomalous beats are aberrantly conducted without convincingly demonstrating a reason for aberrancy* (e.g., right bundle branch block

[RBBB] pattern in a right sided lead, premature P wave, relatively narrow QRS complex).

10. *Forgetting to use more than one monitoring lead* (or to obtain a 12-lead electrocardiogram [ECG]) *for dysrhythmia recognition,* particularly for detecting flutter waves, distinguishing between fine ventricular fibrillation and asystole, and differentiating premature ventricular contractions (PVCs) from aberrancy (morphologic clues).

NEW TRENDS IN THE PHARMACOLOGIC MANAGEMENT OF CARDIAC ARREST

Epinephrine

The importance of epinephrine in the management of cardiac arrest has been known since 1896. More than 80 years later the drug is still regarded as the most useful agent in the pharmacologic treatment of cardiovascular collapse but by a different mechanism than is generally appreciated.

Epinephrine is an endogenous catecholamine with both α- and β-adrenergic properties. In addition to its potent chronotropic and inotropic effect, the α-adrenergic action of epinephrine increases peripheral vascular resistance, which in turn raises diastolic pressure. Since coronary blood flow occurs principally during diastole, this vasoconstrictor effect becomes instrumental in maintaining coronary perfusion while CPR is in progress (Otto et al., 1981; Parmley et al., 1982; Redding, 1979).

Although the recommended dose of epinephrine for treating ventricular fibrillation and asystole is 0.5 to 1.0 mg IV, the smaller dose may be too low. If an initial 1 mg IV bolus of epinephrine proves to be ineffective, one should not forget to repeat the drug at frequent intervals until the desired effect is achieved. If an IV bolus of drug is successful in producing an acceptable blood pressure in a patient with complete heart block or an idioventricular rhythm, an IV infu-

sion of epinephrine may be used to maintain the effect.

Isoproterenol

Isoproterenol is a pure β-adrenergic receptor stimulator with potent chronotropic and inotropic properties. It is indicated for the treatment of hemodynamically significant atropine-resistant bradydysrhythmias when a pacemaker is not readily available. However, its use should be tempered by the arrhythmogenic side effects of the drug, the increase in myocardial oxygen consumption that it causes, and the fact that its β-adrenergic action results in peripheral vasodilation that may impair coronary perfusion by decreasing diastolic blood pressure. Thus when confronted with a patient in asystole or with a hemodynamically significant bradydysrhythmia necessitating CPR, the use of epinephrine seems preferable to isoproterenol (Otto et al., 1981; Parmley et al., 1982; Redding, 1979).

Sodium bicarbonate

Much less sodium bicarbonate is required during cardiac resuscitation than was previously recommended. In cases in which the period of arrest is less than a minute, restoration of adequate ventilation is usually sufficient to correct acidosis, and no sodium bicarbonate is indicated. If the period of arrest is longer, 1 to 2 ampules of sodium bicarbonate may be given depending on the size of the patient and the estimated time since the onset of the arrest. (An initial dose of 1 mEq/kg is usually recommended.)

Adverse effects of excessive sodium bicarbonate administration include extreme alkalosis, hyperosmolality, hypokalemia, sodium overload, shifting of the oxyhemoglobin dissociation curve leftward with consequent impaired oxygen release to the tissues, and precipitation of convulsions and/or arrhythmias. In a hospital setting ABGs assist in determining how much of this drug should be given. Correction of acidosis beyond a pH of 7.25 to 7.30 increases the risk of inducing alkalosis and is probably not warranted.

Bretylium

Bretylium is a quaternary ammonium compound that was initially used in the 1950s as an antihypertensive agent. The drug has a complex mechanism of action including adrenergic stimulation that results in an initial release of norepinephrine followed several minutes later by adrenergic blockade in which the uptake of norepinephrine and epinephrine into adrenergic nerve endings is prevented. This latter effect predominates and accounts for the fact that following an initial increase in blood pressure, hypotension commonly occurs.

Bretylium is useful in the treatment of refractory ventricular fibrillation. The drug exerts an antifibrillation effect that facilitates subsequent electrical conversion. For treatment of ventricular fibrillation, an IV bolus of 5 to 10 mg/kg should be given over 2 minutes. The onset of the action of this drug may be delayed anywhere from 2 to 15 minutes (Dhurandhar et al., 1980; Haynes et al., 1981; Holder et al., 1977) so that resuscitation efforts should not be abandoned until a reasonable period of time is allowed for the drug to take effect. A 10 mg/kg dosage of bretylium may be repeated every 15 to 30 minutes until a maximum of 30 mg/kg is given. If subsequent countershock is successful in converting the patient out of ventricular fibrillation, an IV infusion of either bretylium or lidocaine may be used to prevent recurrence.

Bretylium is also useful in the treatment of refractory ventricular tachycardia; 500 mg is diluted in 50 ml of 5% dextrose in water (D_5W) and infused over a 10-minute period. This can be followed by a continuous infusion.

Bretylium should probably not be used as a first-line agent for the treatment of PVCs, since there is more experience with lidocaine and procainamide in this situation. However, the drug may be useful in treating malignant ventricular arrhythmias that have not responded to lidocaine or procainamide.

Lidocaine

Lidocaine has long been accepted as the antiarrhythmic agent of choice for the treatment of PVCs in the setting of acute ischemia. However, it is only recently that the routine use of this drug has been recommended as a prophylactic measure to prevent primary ventricular fibrillation in patients suspected of having acute infarction even when they do not manifest ventricular ectopy.

Patients at greatest risk of developing ventricular fibrillation with acute myocardial infarction are those seen within the first few hours of the onset of symptoms and in whom a high clinical index of suspicion of infarction exists. This is the group most suited to receive prophylactic treatment with lidocaine. Treatment of patients over 70 years of age is probably not as essential, since the incidence of primary ventricular fibrillation is less in this age group and the risk of toxicity is significantly greater (Goldman et al., 1979; Lie et al., 1974). Lidocaine is useful in the treatment of refractory ventricular fibrillation and is an alternative agent to bretylium in this setting.

Atropine

Atropine is a parasympatholytic agent that has long been used in the treatment of bradydysrhythmias. However, the drug is not without adverse effects; it may produce either atrial or ventricular tachydysrhythmias that increase myocardial oxygen consumption and sometimes precipitate angina. As a result, the clinical indications for atropine should be restricted to bradydysrhythmias that are of hemodynamic significance.

In addition to its vagolytic effect, atropine increases conduction through the AV node. This explains its beneficial effect in the treatment of second- and third-degree AV block during the early hours of acute inferior infarction, when these conduction defects often reflect excessive vagal tone. The drug is not expected to work as well after the first few hours of inferior infarction or with anterior infarction in which excessive parasympathetic tone is less of a causative factor. Because of the fact that certain individuals demonstrate parasympathetic innervation of the ventricles, atropine may occasionally be effective in the treatment of slow idioventricular rhythms or even in asystole.

Calcium chloride

In the past calcium chloride was recommended for the treatment of asystole or EMD. Recent studies suggest that the use of calcium chloride in patients with cardiovascular collapse may be associated with an unfavorable outcome in a significant percentage of patients (Stueven et al., 1983). Whether this is the result of the high serum calcium levels that are routinely induced by the IV administration of the drug (a mean serum calcium level of 15 mg% is recorded following a 500 mg IV bolus to patients in cardiopulmonary arrest) (Dembo, 1981; Resnekov, 1981), or the result of cerebral hypoperfusion secondary to a calcium-induced spasm of the cerebral vasculature (White et al., 1983) is still unknown. Furthermore, preliminary work suggests that the administration of calcium antagonists during arrest improves neurologic recovery (Winegar et al., 1983). Calcium chloride might be expected to produce the opposite effect. At this time, calcium chloride should perhaps only be used in the treatment of asystole or EMD after sodium bicarbonate and repeated doses of epinephrine have been unsuccessful.

Dopamine

Dopamine is a chemical precursor of norepinephrine that exerts dopaminergic as well as α- and β-receptor stimulating actions. Which of these pharmacologic effects predominates depends primarily on the rate of infusion of the drug.

At low infusion rates (1 to 2 μg/kg/min), the dopaminergic effect produces dilation of renal and mesenteric blood vessels. At dosages of 2 to 10 μg/kg/min, the β-receptor stimulating action prevails, resulting in an increase in cardiac output. At dosages greater than 10 μg/kg/min, the α-receptor stimulating effect predominates, causing increased peripheral vasoconstriction that eventually reverses the initial dilation of the renal and mesenteric vasculature.

Dopamine is indicated for the medical treatment of hemodynamically significant hypotension and cardiogenic shock. It is probably the most commonly used pressor agent for this purpose. However, at higher infusion rates (greater than 15 to 20 μg/kg/min) the vasoconstrictor effect predominates, and the action of dopamine resembles that of norepinephrine.

Verapamil

Verapamil has become the pharmacologic agent of choice for the treatment of paroxysmal supraventricular tachycardia (PSVT). This calcium-channel blocking agent exerts its primary effect on AV nodal tissue, slowing conduction and prolonging the effective refractory period within the AV node. As a result, the drug is extremely effective in terminating PSVT by interrupting the reentrant pathway and in slowing the ventricular response to atrial flutter and/ or fibrillation.

PSVT should first be treated by attempting to increase vagal tone with either carotid sinus massage (CSM) (provided there is no evidence of carotid disease) or the Valsalva maneuver. If these vagal maneuvers are not successful, verapamil becomes the drug of choice. The dose is 0.075 to 0.150 mg/kg (usually 5 to 10 mg in an adult) given as an IV bolus over 1 to 2 minutes or over 3 to 4 minutes in the elderly.

Verapamil usually works within minutes and is successful in converting over 90% of the cases of PSVT. Although it only infrequently converts atrial fibrillation or flutter to sinus rhythm, the drug effectively slows the ventricular response to both of these tachydysrhythmias. If the initial dose of verapamil does not produce the desired effect, a second dose (usually 10 mg IV) may be repeated in 30 minutes.

Verapamil may produce a transient reduction

in arterial blood pressure. Because of its depressant effect on sinoatrial (SA) and AV conduction, the drug should be used cautiously in patients with evidence of sinus node disease (sick sinus syndrome [SSS]) or in conjunction with digitalis, which also slows AV nodal conduction. For the same reason verapamil should probably not be administered within 30 minutes of IV propranolol.

Verapamil does *not* have any role in the treatment of ventricular dysrhythmias. The drug should not be used indiscriminately as a diagnostic maneuver and/or therapeutic trial in patients with regular, wide QRS complex tachydysrhythmias in whom ventricular tachycardia is likely to be present, since verapamil may cause ventricular tachycardia to further deteriorate into ventricular fibrillation. Finally, verapamil should not be used to slow the heart rate of a patient in sinus tachycardia in which the rapid heart rate may be needed to sustain cardiac output. Treatment of sinus tachycardia must be directed at the underlying cause.

NEW DEVELOPMENTS IN CPR

In the past it was assumed that the mechanism of blood flow during CPR was the direct result of compressing the heart between the sternum and the vertebral column (cardiac pump theory). In certain individuals with compliant chest walls (especially children), cardiac compression probably does occur to at least some extent, but the observation that repeated forceful coughing during ventricular fibrillation could generate sufficient cardiac output to sustain consciousness (cough CPR) led researchers to believe that other mechanisms might also be operative. Subsequent studies have demonstrated that during CPR cardiac chamber size does not change significantly, pressures remain equal in all cardiac chambers and intrathoracic vessels, and the mitral valve never closes (Bircher, 1982; Luce et al., 1980). If blood flow were simply the result of direct heart compression, one would expect pressures in the left ventricle to dramat-

ically increase as blood was "squeezed" out of this chamber. The mitral valve would close in response to the high pressure gradient produced between the left ventricle and the left atrium, and heart size would decrease as blood was ejected from the aorta.

Instead, the increase in intrathoracic pressure that occurs with external chest compression is generalized. The heart cannot be operating as a pump, since no pressure gradient is developed anywhere within the chest. However, a pressure gradient does develop between the intrathoracic and extrathoracic compartments, and this produces the impetus for the forward (antegrade) flow of blood.

Blood flow with sternal compression is primarily unidirectional out of the aorta. It has been postulated that a valve exists in the jugular vein at the thoracic inlet. Competence of this valve explains why retrograde flow does not occur out of the thoracic cavity. The presence of venous valves elsewhere in the jugular vein is evidenced by the fact that blood does not flow up the neck during a Valsalva maneuver. Whether or not a valve exists precisely at the thoracic inlet is still the subject of much controversy. In any case the lack of retrograde flow out of the thoracic cavity may be explained by the functional closure that occurs when the thinwalled jugular vein is collapsed by the increase in intrathoracic pressure generated by external chest compression. On the other hand, the thick-walled carotid artery remains patent throughout CPR and allows transmission of intrathoracic pressure to the extrathoracic compartment. Extrathoracic venous pressure does not rise significantly during CPR (retrograde flow out of the thorax is prevented), whereas pressure in the carotid artery goes up markedly. The intrathoracic-extrathoracic pressure gradient produced accounts for the principal mechanism of blood flow during CPR, and the heart mainly serves as a conduit for this flow (thoracic pump theory) (Luce et al., 1980; Niemann et al., 1981).

Acceptance of the thoracic pump theory has led researchers to examine whether or not cardiac output during CPR might be enhanced by further increasing intrathoracic pressure. Whereas traditional CPR calls for interposition of ventilations with every fifth cardiac compression, altering this sequence to coordinate external chest compressions simultaneously with ventilation might accomplish this end. This modification in the performance of conventional CPR has been termed *simultaneous compression-ventilation CPR* (SCV-CPR). Intrathoracic pressure is maximized, and studies have shown that peripheral and carotid blood flow are increased by this technique.

Abdominal binding may further increase intrathoracic pressure (Niemann et al., 1982). This procedure exerts its effect by limiting the passive movement of the diaphragm during CPR and/or reducing the size of the vascular compartment. Carotid blood flow goes up, and as a result of the increase in aortic afterload, this augmented blood flow may be preferentially redistributed to the coronary and cerebral vascular beds. Application of military antishock trousers (MAST suit) may result in a similar favorable redistribution of carotid blood flow during CPR (Lilja et al., 1981).

The two final modifications that have been suggested in the performance of conventional CPR are in the rate and duration of external cardiac compressions. Traditionally, a rate of 60 compressions per minute has been recommended for two-rescuer CPR with each compression lasting for 50% of the compression-relaxation cycle. In practice, more attention seems to be directed to complying with the rate criteria. Rescuers may meticulously count off one per second cardiac compressions, often without concentrating on whether they maintain each compression for the required amount of time. In fact, duration of compression is a more important variable to control than is the number of compressions performed per minute. Carotid blood flow increases as the duration of com-

pression increases, and significantly higher antegrade flow can be achieved when compression duration is extended to occupy at least 60% of the compression-relaxation cycle (Luce et al., 1980; Parmley et al., 1982). On the other hand, alteration in the rate of compressions between 40 and 80 times per minute does not significantly affect carotid blood flow (Luce et al., 1980). A more relaxed rate of 40 compressions per minute has been proposed with prolongation of compression duration to 60% of the cycle.

Incorporation of the four modifications just discussed constitutes the "new *CPR*."

- High pressure ventilations simultaneous with compressions (SCV-CPR)
- Abdominal binding
- Slower rate of compression of 40 times per minute
- Prolongation of compression duration to 60% of the compression-relaxation cycle

When pressure in the hypopharynx exceeds 25 cm H_2O, the gastroesophageal sphincter of most patients opens. The resulting gastric insufflation prevents the performance of effective CPR and eventually leads to regurgitation of gastric contents with aspiration. To avoid gastric insufflation, the high pressure ventilation of the new CPR requires endotracheal intubation. Mechanical CPR is probably also required, since fine coordination of ventilation simultaneous with compression and extension of compression duration to 60% of the compression-relaxation cycle are difficult parameters to consistently achieve by human endeavor. Consequently, the new CPR is not yet readily applicable in the field, and until further studies are done to confirm the usefulness of this new technique in a hospital setting, adherence to current standards for two-rescuer CPR should be continued. However, several features of the new CPR should be kept in mind while performing conventional CPR. Since augmentation of carotid blood flow seems to be affected by alteration in the duration of compression but not by changes in rate (between 40 and 80 compressions per minute), more attention should probably be directed to *maintaining compressions for at least 50% of each cycle* rather than preoccupying oneself with rate. In addition, since simultaneous administration of ventilation and compressions increases carotid blood flow, one probably need not be as concerned with strict interposition of ventilation and compression. Instead, concentration on delivering a *full* ventilation should be the goal even if slight asynchrony in CPR results.

Two final questions remain.

1. Does the increased carotid blood flow produced by the new CPR result in improved cerebral perfusion?
2. Is coronary blood flow increased with the new CPR?

Although one might logically assume that the increase in carotid blood flow generated by the techniques just mentioned would naturally improve cerebral perfusion, this is not necessarily the case (Luce et al., 1980). In addition to the cerebral vasculature, the carotid artery also supplies the extracranial circulation. Thus increases in carotid flow may be preferentially distributed away from the brain. Further studies must be done to determine if enhanced carotid flow obtained with the new CPR reflects improved cerebral perfusion.

Second, one must ask what effect this improvement in carotid flow has on coronary perfusion. Since the coronary arteries are primarily perfused during diastole, increasing systolic blood pressure during external chest compression without also increasing diastolic blood pressure would not be expected to improve coronary blood flow (Luce et al., 1980; Niemann et al., 1982). Neither conventional CPR nor SCV-CPR significantly affects diastolic blood pressure. Use of abdominal binding and/or application of the MAST suit may favorably redistribute blood flow to the coronary circulation during CPR, but these techniques are cumbersome to employ during cardiac resuscitation, and their

use cannot be recommended at the present time. Moreover, to encourage the use of the MAST suit or abdominal binding while CPR is being performed on patients in ventricular fibrillation might divert attention and delay treatment of the primary disorder. Electrical countershock must be delivered as soon as the diagnosis of ventricular fibrillation is made. Conversely, pharmacologic therapy with α-adrenergic agents such as epinephrine increases peripheral vascular resistance (and diastolic blood pressure), effectively increasing coronary blood flow during CPR without interrupting the resuscitation process (Otto et al., 1981; Parmley et al., 1982; Redding, 1979). (See new trends in the pharmacologic management of cardiac arrest—epinephrine.)

In summary, new developments in CPR hold promise of significantly increasing carotid blood flow during cardiac resuscitation. Ideally the enhanced carotid blood flow will result in improved cerebral perfusion and better preservation of neurologic function. The addition of pharmacologic agents such as epinephrine is needed to optimize coronary perfusion. Despite these advancements, questions remain regarding the long-term clinical efficacy of the new CPR. For the present, more consideration should probably be given to duration of compression rather than rate and to delivery of full ventilations even if they are not always precisely interposed with compressions. Otherwise current recommendations for the performance of conventional CPR should be followed until more conclusive evidence supports the applicability of the new CPR and a beneficial effect on long-term survival.

INDICATIONS FOR EMERGENCY CARDIAC PACING

Acute myocardial infarction
   Mobitz II second-degree AV block
   Third-degree AV block with anterior myocardial infarction
   New bifascicular bundle branch block

New unifascicular bundle branch block (controversial)

Severe sinus bradycardia ⎫
Mobitz I second-degree AV block ⎬ When hemodynamically significant and resistant to medical therapy
Third-degree AV block with inferior myocardial infarction ⎭

Cardiac arrest
Mobitz II second-degree AV block
Third-degree AV block
Slow idioventricular escape rhythm
Asystole
Severe sinus bradycardia ⎫
Mobitz I second-degree AV block ⎬ When hemodynamically significant and resistant to medical therapy
Refractory tachydysrhythmias including torsade de pointes (overdrive pacing)

DETECTION AND MANAGEMENT OF EMD

EMD is diagnosed when there is evidence of organized electrical activity on an ECG but no effective mechanical contraction (pulselessness). This disorder is most commonly associated with one or more of the following underlying etiologies:

- Inadequate ventilation (intubation of the right mainstem bronchus, tension pneumothorax)
- Pericardial effusion with tamponade
- Myocardial rupture or aortic aneurysm rupture
- Persistent acidosis or other metabolic derangement
- Massive pulmonary embolus
- Hypovolemia (from acute blood loss or septic, neurogenic, or cardiogenic shock)

Although treatment with epinephrine, the appropriate use of sodium bicarbonate, and possibly calcium chloride are recommended, discovery and correction of the causative factor(s) usually offer the only realistic chance for survival.

When confronted with a patient in EMD who has not responded to pharmacologic management, one must rapidly check for adequacy of ventilation. The absence of breath sounds on the left suggests intubation of the right mainstem bronchus. Simply withdrawing the endotracheal tube a small distance should restore bilateral breath sounds. If this maneuver is not successful and/or breath sounds are absent on the right and tracheal deviation is present, the possibility of tension pneumothorax should be considered. One's index of suspicion for tension pneumothorax should be further aroused with significant trauma or in patients with asthma or chronic obstructive pulmonary disease, particularly if they have been on a respirator. If time does not allow for radiographic confirmation, a diagnostic and therapeutic tap with a large-bore needle should be performed in the second or third intercostal space. The needle should be inserted over the top of the rib (to avoid the intercostal vessels that run along the lower border of each rib) and in the midclavicular line (to avoid the internal mammary artery that lies medially). Air under tension produces a hissing sound, and prompt improvement of the patient's hemodynamic condition usually follows.

If inadequate ventilation is not the problem, attention should be directed to assessing volume status. Was the patient dehydrated on admission? Has he gone into cardiogenic shock from a massive myocardial infarction? Was he at risk for throwing a pulmonary embolus? Did he have a known aortic aneurysm? Was his condition septic? Even without an obvious cause of hypovolemia, strong consideration should be given to administration of a fluid challenge at this point.

Other potentially reversible causes of EMD in a hospitalized patient include persistent acidosis (diabetic ketoacidosis, lactic acidosis), electrolyte disturbance (hyperkalemia, hypokalemia), and pericardial effusion with tamponade. Obtaining ABGs and serum electrolyte concentrations will help investigate the first two possibilities. If tamponade is suggested by either the history (uremia, pericarditis, fractured ribs from too vigorous CPR) and/or the physical examination (jugular venous distention, muffled heart sounds), pericardiocentesis should be performed. Withdrawing as little as 50 ml of fluid under these circumstances may be lifesaving.

Emergency pericardiocentesis is best performed through a subxiphoid approach with insertion of the needle at a 20° to 30° angle with the frontal plane. The needle should be directed toward the tip of the left shoulder, and aspiration should be continuous. Entry into the pericardium usually produces a distinct "giving" sensation that should be followed by the appearance of nonclotting blood into the syringe. If the blood clots, it most likely has been removed from the right ventricle.

When time does not permit the use of ECG monitoring from the pericardiocentesis needle, the chance of causing epicardial injury may be minimized by using a 20-gauge spinal needle as an exploring needle over which a larger-bore needle has been threaded. Once the pericardial sac has been entered with the spinal needle, drainage may be accomplished by advancing the large-bore needle and then removing the spinal needle.

Two additional measures that may be helpful in improving cardiac output while preparation for pericardiocentesis is being made or in the event that pericardiocentesis is unsuccessful are fluid challenge and isoproterenol infusion. Rapid administration of fluid increases left ventricular filling pressure and augments stroke volume. Isoproterenol increases heart rate and myocardial contractility but lowers systemic vascular resistance. This results in enhanced cardiac output in the presence of cardiac tamponade. Treatment of EMD with isoproterenol under these circumstances is preferable to using other pressor agents (dopamine, epinephrine) that might increase peripheral vascular resistance and impede forward stroke volume.

Finally, EMD that occurs with trauma should prompt the emergency care provider to actively consider an alternative set of causes. The mechanism of injury may be enlightening. Learning that a victim's automobile was demolished in a high-speed freeway accident in which the patient's chest deformed the steering wheel before his head crashed through the windshield should suggest at least four possible etiologies to explain EMD including the following:
- Acute blood loss (internal hemorrhage from abdominal injury, pelvic fracture, etc.)
- Cardiogenic shock from myocardial contusion (the result of the steering wheel injury)
- Neurogenic shock from cervical spine injury
- Pericardial tamponade, bilateral pneumothorax, or tension pneumothorax from trauma to the chest wall

SUGGESTED READINGS

American Heart Association Subcommittee on Emergency Cardiac Care: Standards and guidelines for cardiopulmonary resuscitation (CPR) and emergency cardiac care (ECC), JAMA 244:453-509, 1980.

Auerbach, P.S., and Budassi, S.A., editors: Cardiac arrest and CPR, Rockville, Md., 1983, Aspen Systems Corp.

Bircher, N.: New concepts in cardiopulmonary resuscitation, ER Reports 3:45-48, 1982.

Dalsey, W.C., Barsan, W.G., Joyce, S.M., Hedges, J.R., Lukes, S.J., and Doan, L.A.: Comparison of superior vena cava vs inferior vena cava access for delivery of drugs using a radioisotope technique during normal perfusion and CPR (abstract), Ann. Emerg. Med. 12:247-248, 1983.

Dembo, D.H.: Calcium in advanced life support, Crit. Care Med. 9:358-359, 1981.

Dhurandhar, R.W., Pickron, J., and Goldman, A.M.: Bretylium tosylate in the management of recurrent ventricular fibrillation complicating acute myocardial infarction, Heart Lung 9:265-270, 1980.

Frank, S.: Cardiopulmonary resuscitation and advanced cardiac life support: common errors and current techniques, J. Fam. Prac. 12:213-217, 1981.

Goldman, L., and Batsford, W.F.: Risk-benefit stratification as a guide to lidocaine prophylaxis of primary ventricular fibrillation in acute myocardial infarction: an analytic review, Yale J. Biol. Med. **52**:455-466, 1979.

Grauer, K.: Should prophylactic lidocaine be routinely used in patients suspected of acute myocardial infarction? J. Fla. Med. Assoc. **69**:377-379, 1982.

Greenberg, M.I., Mayeda, D.V., Chrzanowski, R., Brumwell, D., Baskin, S.I., and Roberts, J.R.: Endotracheal administration of atropine sulfate, Ann. Emerg. Med. **11**:546-548, 1982.

Haynes, R.E., Chinn, T.L., Copass, M.K., and Cobb, L.A.: Comparison of bretylium tosylate and lidocaine in management of out of hospital ventricular fibrillation: a randomized clinical trial, Am. J. Cardiol. **48**:353-356, 1981.

Holder, D.A., Sniderman, A.D., Fraser, G., and Fallen, E.L.: Experience with bretylium tosylate by a hospital cardiac arrest team, Circulation **55**:541-544, 1977.

Kuhn, G.J., White, B.C., Swetnam, R.E., Mumey, J.F., Rydesky, M.F., Tintinalli, J.E., Krome, R.L., and Hoehner, P.J.: Peripheral vs central circulation times during CPR: a pilot study, Ann. Emerg. Med. **10**:417-419, 1981.

Lie, K.I., Wellens, H.J., van Capelle, F.J., and Durrer, D.: Lidocaine in prevention of primary ventricular fibrillation, New Engl. J. Med. **291**:1324-1326, 1974.

Lilja, G.P., Long, R.S., and Ruiz, E.: Augmentation of systolic blood pressure during external cardiac compression by use of the MAST suit, Ann. Emerg. Med. **10**:182-184, 1981.

Luce, J.M., Cary, J.M., Ross, B.K., Culver, B.H., and Butler, J.: New developments in cardiopulmonary resuscitation, JAMA **244**:1366-1370, 1980.

McIntyre, K.M., Parisi, A.F., Benfari, R., Goldberg, A.H., and Dalen, J.E.: Pathophysiologic syndromes of cardiopulmonary resuscitation, Arch. Intern. Med. **138**:1130-1133, 1978.

McIntyre, K.M., and Lewis, J.A., editors: Textbook of advanced cardiac life support, Dallas, 1981, American Heart Association.

Moncure, A.C., and McEnany, M.T.: Cardiovascular emergencies. In Wilkins, E.W., editor: MGH textbook of emergency medicine, Baltimore, 1978, The Williams & Wilkins Co., pp. 377-381.

Niemann, J.T., Rosborough, J., Hausknecht, M., Ung, S., and Criley, J.M.: Blood flow without cardiac compression during closed chest CPR, Crit. Care Med. **9**:380-381, 1981.

Niemann, J.T., Rosborough, J.P., Ung, S., and Criley, J.M.: Coronary perfusion pressure during experimental cardiopulmonary resuscitation, Ann. Emerg. Med. **11**:127-131, 1982.

Otto, C.W., Yakaitis, R.W., and Blitt, C.D.: Mechanism of action of epinephrine in resuscitation from asphyxial arrest, Crit. Care Med. **9**:321-324, 1981.

Parmley, W.W., Hatcher, C.R., Ewy, G.A., Furman, S., Redding, J., and Weisfeldt, M.L.: Task Force V: physical interventions and adjunctive therapy, Thirteenth Bethesda Conference on Emergency Cardiac Care, Am. J. Cardiol. **50**:409-420, 1982.

Redding, J.S.: Cardiopulmonary resuscitation: an algorithm and some common pitfalls, Am. Heart J. **98**:788-797, 1979.

Redding, J.S.: Commentary on the proceedings: Second Wolf Creek Conference on CPR, Crit. Care Med. **9**:432-435, 1981.

Resnekov, L.: Calcium antagonist drugs—myocardial preservation and reduced vulnerability to ventricular fibrillation during CPR, Crit. Care Med. **9**:360-361, 1981.

Rogers, M.C.: New developments in cardiopulmonary resuscitation, Pediatrics **71**:655-658, 1983.

Safar, P.: Cardiopulmonary cerebral resuscitation, Stavanger, Norway, 1981, Asmund S. Laerdal.

Stueven, H., Thompson, B.M., Aprahamian, C., and Darin, J.C.: Use of calcium in prehospital cardiac arrest, Ann. Emerg. Med. **12**:136-139, 1983.

Weaver, W.D., Cobb, L.A., Compass, M.K., and Hallstrom, A.P.: Ventricular defibrillation—a comparative trial using 175-J and 320-J shocks, N. Engl. J. Med. **307**:1101-1106, 1982.

White, B.C., Winegar, C.D., Wilson, R.F., Hoehner, P.J., and Trombley, J.H.: Possible role of calcium blockers in cerebral resuscitation: a review of the literature and synthesis for future studies, Crit. Care Med. **11**:202-207, 1983.

Winegar, C.P., Henderson, O., White, B.C., Jackson, R.E., O'Hara, T., Krause, G.S., Vigor, D.N., Kontry, R., Wilson, W., and Shelby-Lane, C.: Early amelioration of neurologic deficit by lidoflazine after fifteen minutes of cardiopulmonary arrest in dogs, Ann. Emerg. Med. **12**:471-477, 1983.

Wyman, M.G., and Gore, S.: Lidocaine prophylaxis in myocardial infarction: a concept whose time has come, Heart Lung **12**:358-361, 1983.

CHAPTER 3

Drug compendium

DRUG CATEGORIES FREQUENTLY USED IN EMERGENCY CARDIAC CARE

Agents for cardiac arrest	Antiarrhythmic agents	Agents for myocardial infarction and/or shock
Epinephrine	Lidocaine	Morphine sulfate
Sodium bicarbonate	Procainamide	Sodium nitroprusside
Atropine sulfate	Bretylium tosylate	Nitroglycerin
Oxygen	Digoxin	Dopamine
Isoproterenol	Verapamil	Dobutamine
Calcium chloride	Propranolol	Norepinephrine

Table 3-1. Emergency cardiac drug index

Drug	Amount per dispensing unit	Mechanism of action	Indications	Dose and routes of administration	Comments
Epinephrine (Adrenalin) (1:10,000 dilution)	1 mg per 10 ml syringe	An endogenous catecholamine with α- and β-receptor stimulating effects Increases automaticity, rate, and force of myocardial contractions Increases systemic vascular resistance and arterial blood pressure	Ventricular fibrillation Asystole EMD Slow idioventricular rhythm and other bradydysrhythmias with hemodynamically significant hypotension (epinephrine infusion)	0.5-1.0 mg IV (5-10 ml of a 1:10,000 solution)—may repeat every 5 min as needed *Begin infusion at 1 μg/min: Mix 1 mg in 250 ml D$_5$W and begin drip at 15 drops/min* Range of infusion = 1-4 μg/min May be given by ET tube or by intracardiac injection (1 mg)	Vasoconstrictor rather than inotropic effect of epinephrine is probably the more important action during cardiac arrest; diastolic blood pressure is increased, and coronary blood flow is favored Administration of 1 mg at more frequent intervals than every 5 min may be needed with cardiovascular collapse Epinephrine is rapidly absorbed across bronchotracheal structures following intratracheal administration Intracardiac injection is fraught with hazard and should only be resorted to when all else fails

ACLS, Advanced cardiac life support.
BLS, Basic life support.
CHF, Congestive heart failure.
COPD, Chronic obstructive pulmonary disease.
D$_5$W, 5% dextrose in water.
ET, Endotracheal tube.

PAT, Paroxysmal atrial tachycardia.
PSVT, Paroxysmal supraventricular tachycardia.
SA, Sinoatrial.
V FIB, Ventricular fibrillation.
VT, Ventricular tachycardia.
WPW, Wolff-Parkinson-White

Table 3-1. Emergency cardiac drug index—cont'd

Drug	Amount per dispensing unit	Mechanism of action	Indications	Dose and routes of administration	Comments
Sodium bicarbonate	50 mEq per 50 ml syringe	Reverse acidosis	Metabolic acidosis from hypoxia and buildup of lactic acid Treatment probably *not* needed with pH $\geq$ 7.25-7.30	Initial dose: 1mEq/kg (about 1-1½ ampules) Subsequent doses are ideally governed by results of ABGs When ABGs are not available, ½ initial dose may be repeated every 10 min	Sodium bicarbonate is *not* usually needed in cases of witnessed arrest when BLS and ACLS are promptly initiated IV line must be thoroughly flushed after giving sodium bicarbonate, since many drugs are inactivated in an alkaline medium Caution against overcorrection of acidosis (iatrogenic metabolic alkalosis) that is difficult to reverse, and may be associated with the following adverse effects: • hyperosmolality • hypokalemia • sodium overload • impaired oxygen release to the tissues • dysrhythmias • seizures

Continued.

Table 3-1. Emergency cardiac drug index—cont'd

Drug	Amount per dispensing unit	Mechanism of action	Indications	Dose and routes of administration	Comments
Atropine sulfate	1 mg per 10 ml syringe	Parasympatholytic action that decreases vagal tone, increases rate of SA nodal discharge, and improves AV conduction	Sinus bradycardia with hypotension and/or PVCs AV block when accompanied by bradycardia and hypotension Slow idioventricular rhythm Asystole	0.5 mg IV every 5 min to a maximum dose of 2 mg (1.0 mg of atropine may be given at a time for marked bradycardia and/or hypotension) May be given by ET tube in same dose	Atropine may occasionally help in asystole when excessive parasympathetic tone is the cause Asymptomatic sinus bradycardia should *not* be treated with atropine Adverse effects include precipitation of atrial or ventricular tachydysrhythmias and a consequent increase in myocardial oxygen consumption
Oxygen	—	Increases oxygen delivery to tissues	Suspected hypoxemia of any cause (cardiopulmonary arrest, myocardial infarction, etc.)	Nasal cannula: 25%-40% O_2 can be delivered with flow rates of 6 L/min Face mask: 50%-60% O_2 can be delivered with flow rates of 10 L/min Venturi mask: Fixed O_2 concentrations of 24%, 28%, 35%, and 40% may be delivered with flow rates of 4-8 L/min Pocket mask: 50% O_2 can be delivered with flow rates of 10 L/min	Oxygen should *never* be withheld for fear of causing CO_2 retention during an emergency cardiac situation

Table 3-1. Emergency cardiac drug index—cont'd

Drug	Amount per dispensing unit	Mechanism of action	Indications	Dose and routes of administration	Comments
Oxygen—cont'd				Bag-valve-mask devices: May deliver room air or up to 90% O_2 with an oxygen source and attached reservoir	
Isoproterenol (Isuprel)	1 mg vials	Synthetic sympathomimetic amine with nearly pure β-adrenergic properties	Hemodynamically significant sinus bradycardia and AV block unresponsive to atropine. Slow idioventricular rhythm	*Begin infusion at 2 µg/min: Mix 1 mg in 250 ml of D_5W and begin drip at 30 drops/min* — Titrate infusion to 20 µg/min depending on heart rate and rhythm response	Increases myocardial oxygen consumption and may produce serious ventricular dysrhythmias, so that one should titrate to lowest possible infusion rate. Use in AV block is usually a temporary stopgap measure until a pacemaker can be inserted. Vasodilatory effect may aggravate existing hypotension in bradydysrhythmias; not recommended in cardiovascular collapse (EMD, asystole) because of its detrimental effect on coronary flow
Calcium chloride (10% solution)	1000 mg (13.6 mEq of calcium per 10 ml syringe)	Increases the myocardial force of contraction	Asystole and EMD; after appropriate doses of epinephrine and sodium bicarbonate	500 mg (5 ml) IV bolus; may repeat once in 10 min	Efficacy in cardiovascular collapse is under investigation; probably should not be used until other agents have been tried and have failed

Continued.

Table 3-1. Emergency cardiac drug index—cont'd

Drug	Amount per dispensing unit	Mechanism of action	Indications	Dose and routes of administration	Comments
Calcium chloride (10% solution)—cont'd					May produce bradycardia or ventricular standstill if given too fast or in excess Serum calcium levels are markedly elevated following administration of an IV bolus of calcium Should be used cautiously in patients taking digitalis, since calcium may precipitate digitalis toxicity
Lidocaine	IV bolus: 100 mg per 10 ml syringe Infusion: 1 g per 25 ml syringe	Elevates ventricular fibrillation threshold Decreases automatically by depressing spontaneous rate of diastolic depolarization Shortens refractory period Has little effect on conduction velocity	Drug of choice for ventricular dysrhythmias occurring during cardiac resuscitation Consider *prophylactic* use for suspected acute myocardial infarction if 1. High index of suspicion for infarction 2. Less than 24 hr since onset of symptoms 3. Patient less than 70 yr old	Initial IV bolus: 1 mg/kg (50-100 mg) May repeat 50-75 mg boluses every 5-10 min up to total loading dose of 225 mg *Begin infusion at 2 mg/min (immediately following initial IV bolus)* *Mix 2 g in 500 ml of D_5W and begin drip at 30 drops/min* Range of infusion = ½-4 mg/min May give 100 mg bolus by ET tube	Begin drug prophylactically in cardiac resuscitation immediately following conversion from V FIB to normal rhythm Use lower infusion rates (½-1 mg/min) for patients with CHF, shock, lower body weight, the elderly, and with concomitant use of propranolol or cimetidine Suspect toxicity if • slurring of speech • paresthesias • confusion • hypotension • seizures

Table 3-1. Emergency cardiac drug index—cont'd

Drug	Amount per dispensing unit	Mechanism of action	Indications	Dose and routes of administration	Comments
Procainamide (Pronestyl)	IV bolus: 100 mg per ml; 10 ml vials Infusion: 1 g per 2 ml vial	Quinidine-like action that slows electrical conduction, increases refractory period, and decreases automaticity by depressing spontaneous rate of diastolic depolarization	Ventricular dysrhythmias	Administer increments of 100 mg IV *slowly* over a 5 min period until 1. The dysrhythmia is controlled 2. A total loading dose of 1 g is given 3. Adverse effects (widening of QRS complex or hypotension) May follow with IV infusion at rate of 1-4 mg/min (prepare infusion in a similar manner as for lidocaine)	Second drug of choice for treating ventricular dysrhythmias when lidocaine is ineffective Also effective against atrial dysrhythmias Alternate IV loading regimen is to infuse 500-1000 mg over 30 min
Bretylium tosylate (Bretylol)	500 mg per 10 ml ampule	Quaternary ammonium compound with complex actions Elevates ventricular fibrillation threshhold Initially releases catecholamines (may cause initial hypertension) Later exerts postganglionic adrenergic blocking effect (may cause hypotension)	Refractory ventricular dysrhythmias	V FIB: 5-10 mg/kg IV bolus (about 500 mg [1 ampule]) May repeat every 15-30 min to maximum total dose of 30 mg/kg VT: Dilute 500 mg in 50 ml of D_5W, and infuse over 10 min May follow loading dose for either V FIB or VT with IV infusion at rate of 1-2 mg/min (prepare infusion in a similar manner as for lidocaine)	Probably is drug of choice (over lidocaine) for refractory V FIB; rarely effects spontaneous conversion of V FIB, but facilitates conversion to normal rhythm with subsequent countershock Should *not* be used as first-line agent for simple PVC suppression Onset of antiarrhythmic effect may be delayed for up to 15 min so that resuscita-

Continued.

Table 3-1. Emergency cardiac drug index—cont'd

Drug	Amount per dispensing unit	Mechanism of action	Indications	Dose and routes of administration	Comments
Bretylium tosylate (Bretylol)—cont'd					tion effort should *not* be terminated prematurely once decision is made to use the drug Postural hypotension is most common adverse effect
Digoxin	IV use: 0.5 mg per 2 ml ampule Oral use: Tablets of 0.250 mg or 0.125 mg	Increases force and velocity of myocardial contraction Prolongs refractory period of AV node by direct effect and enhancement of vagal tone; thus slows ventricular response to supraventricular tachydysrhythmias	Atrial fibrillation/flutter with rapid ventricular response Indications limited in emergency cardiac setting Second drug of choice after verapamil for PSVT	*For patients not previously digitalized:* 0.25-0.50 mg IV initially May follow with 0.125-0.250 mg IV increments every 2-6 hr to a total of 0.75-1.50 mg over the first 24 hr; this schedule can be adjusted according to the ventricular response	Use cautiously with acute ischemia, COPD, hypokalemia, or hypercalcemia Avoid cardioversion if possible in patients receiving digoxin Suspect digitalis toxicity with • nausea, vomiting • disturbances of color vision (uncommon) • recent addition of quinidine • recent worsening of renal function • presence of certain cardiac dysrhythmias such as frequent PVCs (especially if multifocal), PAT with block, junctional tachycardia, Wenckebach rhythms,

Table 3-1. Emergency cardiac drug index—cont'd

Drug	Amount per dispensing unit	Mechanism of action	Indications	Dose and routes of administration	Comments
Digoxin—cont'd					slow atrial fibrillation Contraindicated for atrial fibrillation with WPW syndrome
Verapamil (Isoptin)	5 mg per 2 ml ampule	Slow channel calcium blocking agent Slows conduction and prolongs refractoriness in AV node Terminates re-entrant tachydysrhythmias and slows ventricular response to atrial fibrillation/flutter	PSVT Atrial fibrillation/flutter with rapid ventricular response	Initial dose: 5-10 mg (0.075-0.150 mg/kg) IV given over a 1-2 min period (or over 3-4 min in the elderly) May repeat once in 30 min if needed	Drug of choice for PSVT (successful conversion to sinus rhythm in over 90% of cases) Effectively slows rate of rapid atrial fibrillation/flutter, but IV form has short duration of action Do not use concomitantly with IV propranolol
Propranolol (Inderal)	1 mg per 1 ml vial	β-Adrenergic receptor blocking agent Decreases automaticity, reduces sinus rate, and prolongs AV conduction time	Refractory ventricular dysrhythmias (useful with digitalis toxicity) Supraventricular tachydysrhythmias Indications limited in emergency cardiac setting	1 mg IV *slowly* over a 5 min period May repeat in 1 mg increments up to total dose of 5 mg	Contraindications: bronchospasm, significant CHF, AV block Do not use concomitantly with IV verapamil
Morphine sulfate	—	Analgesic action Increases venous capacitance, thus	Pain and anxiety of acute ischemic chest pain Acute left ventricular failure with	2-5 mg IV; may repeat every 5-30 min as needed	Cautious dosing by giving small IV increments at frequent intervals is advised

Continued.

Table 3-1. Emergency cardiac drug index—cont'd

Drug	Amount per dispensing unit	Mechanism of action	Indications	Dose and routes of administration	Comments
Morphine sulfate—cont'd		decreasing venous return Reduces systemic vascular resistance	pulmonary edema		Excessive use of this drug may cause bradycardia, hypotension, oversedation, nausea, or respiratory depression Respiratory depression may be reversed with 0.4 mg IV naloxone (Narcan); other vagotonic actions may be reversed by atropine
Sodium nitroprusside (Nipride)	50 mg per 5 ml vial	Direct peripheral vasodilator *both* of arterial (decreases afterload) and venous (decreases preload) systems	Hypertensive crisis Treatment of complications of acute myocardial infarction: • hypertension • left ventricular failure	Begin infusion at 10 µg/min: Mix 50 mg in 250 ml of D_5W and begin drip at 3 drops/min Range of infusion = 0.5-8.0 µg/kg/min May increase infusion rate by 3 drops/min (10 µg/min) every 5 min Minute-to-minute titration of dose is required	Use of this drug for left ventricular failure in acute myocardial infarction usually requires invasive hemodynamic monitoring Cover IV bottle with aluminum foil because of sensitivity to light Thiocyanate toxicity (tinnitus, blurred vision, delirium) should be watched for if large doses are used, if the duration of treatment is long, and/or the patient has renal failure
Nitroglycerin	Tablets for sublingual use: 0.3 mg (1/	Vascular smooth muscle relaxant Selectively di-	Sublingual, topical form: Drug of choice for acute ischemic	Sublingual: 0.3-0.4 mg every 3-5 min up to three times	Main side effects of sublingual and topical forms of drug are head-

Table 3-1. Emergency cardiac drug index—cont'd

Drug	Amount per dispensing unit	Mechanism of action	Indications	Dose and routes of administration	Comments
Nitroglycerin —cont'd	200 gr) 0.4 mg (1/ 150 gr) 0.6 mg (1/ 100 gr) IV use: Prepared by pharmacy (not yet commercially available)	lates coronary arteries Produces predominant venodilation (decreases preload) with a lesser reduction of peripheral vascular resistance	chest pain (angina, coronary spasm, myocardial infarction) IV infusion: Treatment of complications of acute myocardial infarction: • persistent chest pain • hypertension • left ventricular failure	Ointment: Apply ½-2 inches every 3-6 hr *IV infusion: Infusion range and rate similar to that for sodium nitroprusside (see above)*	ache and hypotension IV use of drug usually requires invasive hemodynamic monitoring IV infusion of nitroglycerin theoretically less likely to produce "coronary steal" than IV nitroprusside
Dopamine (Intropin)	200 mg per 5 ml ampule	Catecholamine precursor of norepinephrine with dopaminergic, α- and β-adrenergic receptor stimulating actions	Cardiogenic shock Hemodynamically significant hypotension	*Begin infusion at about 400 µg/ min: Mix 200 mg in 250 ml of D_5W and begin drip at 30 drops/min* Titrate drip upward and adjust for lowest infusion rate that maintains desired clinical response	May cause tachydysrhythmias, necessitating reduction of infusion rate Effects of dopamine dose-related: *1-2 µg/kg/min*— dilates renal and mesenteric blood vessels (dopaminergic effect) *2-10 µg/kg/min*— exerts predominant β-adrenergic stimulating effect that increases cardiac output *10-20 µg/kg/min*— exerts predominant α-adrenergic stimulating effect that results in peripheral vasoconstriction *>20 µg/kg/min*— may reverse the dilation of renal and mesenteric blood vessels

Continued.

Table 3-1. Emergency cardiac drug index—cont'd

Drug	Amount per dispensing unit	Mechanism of action	Indications	Dose and routes of administration	Comments
Dobutamine (Dobutrex)	250 mg per 20 ml vial	Synthetic catecholamine with predominantly β-adrenergic receptor stimulating actions	Cardiogenic shock	*Begin infusion at 250 μg/min: Mix 250 mg in 250 ml of D_5W and begin drip at 15 drops/min* Range of infusion = 2.5-10.0 μg/kg/min Titrate drip upward and adjust for lowest infusion rate that maintains desired clinical response	Dobutamine improves myocardial contractility while producing only minimal vasoconstriction and little change in heart rate; also less arrhythmogenic than dopamine (dopamine may be preferable for severe heart failure with frank hypotension as a result of its greater vasoconstrictor properties)
Norepinephrine (Levophed)	8 mg per ampule	Endogenous catecholamine with both α- and β-receptor stimulating *effects* (most potent of the vasopressors)	Cardiogenic shock Hemodynamically significant hypotension	*Begin infusion at 2-3 μg/min: Mix ½ ampule (4 mg) in 250 ml of D_5W (= 16 μg/ml) and begin drip at about 10 drops/min* Titrate drip upward and adjust for lowest infusion rate that maintains desired clinical response	Usually reserved for treatment of shock that has not responded to other agents May compromise renal and mesenteric blood flow Extravasation from peripheral IV may cause sloughing of superficial tissues

Table 3-2. Commonly used drugs and doses in resuscitation of children compared to adults

Drug	Dosing regimen	Weight of patient	Recommended dose	
Atropine sulfate	Child 0.01 mg/kg Adult 0.5 mg IV every 5 min to 2 mg	10 kg 20 kg 30 kg Adult	0.1 mg IV 0.2 mg IV 0.3 mg IV 0.5 mg IV	
Epinephrine	Child 0.01 mg/kg Adult 0.5-1.0 mg IV (i.e., 5-10 ml of 1:10,000 solution)	10 kg 20 kg 30 kg Adult	0.1 mg (1 ml) IV 0.2 mg (2 ml) IV 0.3 mg (3 ml) IV 0.5-1 mg (5-10 ml) IV	
Calcium chloride (10% solution)	Child 0.1 ml/kg Adult 500 mg (5 ml); may repeat in 10 min	10 kg 20 kg 30 kg Adult	100 mg (1 ml) IV 200 mg (2 ml) IV 300 mg (3 ml) IV 500 mg (5 ml) IV	
Sodium bicarbonate	Child 1 mEq/kg Adult 1 mEq/kg initially; repeat ½ this dose every 10 min	10 kg 20 kg 30 kg Adult	10 mEq (⅓ ampule) IV 20 mEq (⅔ ampule) IV 30 mEq (⅗ ampule) IV 50-100 mEq (1-2 ampules) IV	
Isoproterenol	Child Begin with 0.1 μg/kg/min Adult 2-20 μg/min infusion range	10 kg 20 kg 30 kg Adult	1 μg/min 2 μg/min 2 μg/min 2 μg/min	Initial drip concentration
Lidocaine	Child 1 mg/kg IV bolus; 20-50 μg/kg/min infusion rate Adult 1 mg/kg IV bolus; 1-4 mg/min infusion rate	10 kg 20 kg 30 kg Adult	*Bolus* 10 mg IV 20 mg IV 30 mg IV 50-100 mg IV	*IV Infusion* 200-500 μg/min 400-1000 μg/min 600-1500 μg/min 1-4 mg/min (1000-4000 μg/min

Continued.

Table 3-2. Commonly used drugs and doses in resuscitation of children compared to adults—cont'd

Drug	Dosing regimen	Weight of patient	Recommended dose
Bretylium	Child	10 kg	50 mg IV bolus
	5 mg/kg IV bolus	20 kg	100 mg IV bolus
	Adult	30 kg	150 mg IV bolus
	5-10 mg/kg IV bolus (i.e., about 500 mg)	Adult	500 mg IV bolus
Defibrillation	Child	10 kg	20 J, then 40 J
	2J/kg, then 4 J/kg	20 kg	40 J, then 80 J
	Adult	30 kg	60 J, then 120 J
	200-300 J two times, then 360 J	Adult	200 J two times, then 360 J
Oxygen	Inadequate oxygenation (hypoxia) produced by respiratory arrest is the most common cause of cardiac arrest in children		

CALCULATION OF IV INFUSION RATES

PROBLEM: Make up a lidocaine infusion. How fast should the drip be set to infuse 2 mg of lidocaine per minute?

ANSWER: Mix 2 g of lidocaine in 500 ml of D_5W.

$$\frac{2\ g}{500\ ml}\left(\text{or}\ \frac{1\ g}{250\ ml}\right) = \frac{4\ g}{1000\ ml} = \frac{4000\ mg}{1000\ ml} = \frac{4\ mg}{ml}\left(=\frac{2\ mg}{\frac{1}{2}\ ml}\right)$$

This gives a concentration of 4 mg of lidocaine per milliliter (or 2 mg of lidocaine per ½ ml).

To run an infusion at a rate of 2 mg/min implies that ½ ml/min of lidocaine must be infused.

> *1 ml = 60 drops for a microdrip*
> (½ ml per min = 30 drops/min)

Set the infusion at a rate of 30 drops/min.

A rate of 15 drops/min infuses 1 mg./min of lidocaine.

A rate of 30 drops/min infuses 2 mg/min of lidocaine.

A rate of 45 drops/min infuses 3 mg/min of lidocaine.

A rate of 60 drops/min infuses 4 mg/min of lidocaine.

• • •

PROBLEM: Make up a procainamide infusion.

ANSWER: Same method as for lidocaine.
Mix 2 g of procainamide in 500 ml of D_5W and set the drip to run at 30 drops/min to infuse 2 mg/min.

• • •

PROBLEM: Make up a bretylium infusion.

ANSWER: Same method as for lidocaine.

Mix 2 g of bretylium in 500 ml of D_5W, and set the drip to run at 30 drops/min to infuse 2 mg/min. (Usually one begins a bretylium infusion at 15 drops/min, which equals 1 mg/min.)

• • •

PROBLEM: Make up an isoproterenol infusion. How fast should the drip be set to achieve an initial infusion rate of 2 μg/min?

ANSWER: Mix 1 mg (1 vial) of isoproterenol in 250 ml of D_5W.

$$\frac{1 \text{ mg}}{250 \text{ ml}} = \frac{4 \text{ mg}}{1000 \text{ ml}} = \frac{4000 \text{ μg}}{1000 \text{ ml}} = \frac{4 \text{ μg}}{\text{ml}} \left(= \frac{2 \text{ μg}}{\frac{1}{2} \text{ ml}} \right)$$

This gives a concentration of 4 μg of isoproterenol per ml (or 2 μg of isoproterenol per ½ ml).

To begin an infusion at a rate of 2 μg/min, ½ ml/min must be infused. Begin drip at a rate of 30 drops/min.

• • •

PROBLEM: Make up an epinephrine infusion.

ANSWER: Same method as for isoproterenol.

Mix 1 mg of epinephrine in 250 ml of D_5W, and set the drip to run at 30 drops/min to infuse 2 μg/min. (Usually one begins an epinephrine infusion at 15 drops/min, which equals 1 μg/min.)

• • •

PROBLEM: Make up a dopamine infusion. How fast should the drip be set to achieve an initial rate of 5 μg/kg/min?

ANSWER: Mix 200 mg (1 ampule) of dopamine in 250 ml of D_5W.

$$\frac{200 \text{ mg}}{250 \text{ ml}} = \frac{800 \text{ mg}}{1000 \text{ ml}} = \frac{800,000 \text{ μg}}{1000 \text{ ml}} = \frac{800 \text{ μg}}{\text{ml}} \left(= \frac{400 \text{ μg}}{\frac{1}{2} \text{ ml}} \right)$$

This gives a concentration of 800 μg of dopamine per ml (or 400 μg of dopamine per ½ ml).

Dopamine exerts its most beneficial effects at an infusion rate of 2 to 10 μg/kg/min. Beginning the infusion rate at an even 5 μg/kg/min, an 80 kg patient would require 400 μg/min (i.e., 5 × 80), which equals ½ ml min that must be infused.

Begin the infusion rate at 30 drops/min.

• • •

An easy way to remember how to prepare IV infusions for the drugs most commonly used during cardiac arrest is to apply the "Rule of 250 ml."

> *Rule of 250 ml:* Mix 1 unit of drug in 250 ml of D_5W, and set the infusion to run at 30 drops/min.*

---

*The Rule of 250 ml depends on the amount of drug contained in one unit. The contents of a vial or an ampule may vary slightly from one hospital to the next so that you need to be familiar with the drug formulary used in your hospital. Calculations in this section assume the following:

1 g of lidocaine
1 g of procainamide } = 1 unit of drug
1 g of bretylium

1 mg (1 vial) of isoproterenol
1 mg (1 ampule) of epinephrine } = 1 unit of drug

200 mg (1 ampule) of dopamine} = 1 unit of drug

Examples:

Lidocaine—Mix 1 g in 250 ml D_5W (or 2 g in 500 ml), and set drip at 30 drops/min to infuse 2 mg/min.

Procainamide—Mix 1 g in 250 ml D_5W (or 2 g in 500 ml), and set drip at 30 drops/min to infuse 2 mg/min.

Bretylium—Mix 1 g in 250 ml D_5W (or 2 g in 500 ml), and set drip at 30 drops/min to infuse 2 mg/min.

Isoproterenol—Mix 1 mg in 250 ml D_5W, and set drip at 30 drops/min to infuse 2 μg/min.

Epinephrine—Mix 1 mg in 250 D_5W, and set drip at 30 drops/min to infuse 2 μg/min.

Dopamine—Mix 200 mg (1 ampule) in 250 ml D_5W, and set drip at 30 drops/min to infuse about 5 μg/kg/min (400 μg/min for an 80 kg patient).

• • •

PROBLEM: Make up a dobutamine infusion. How fast should the drip be set to achieve an initial infusion rate of 2.5 μg/kg/min with an 80 kg patient?

ANSWER: Mix 250 mg (1 vial) of dobutamine in 250 ml of D_5/W.

$$\frac{250 \text{ mg}}{250 \text{ ml}} = \frac{1000 \text{ mg}}{1000 \text{ ml}} = \frac{1 \text{ mg}}{1 \text{ ml}} = \frac{1000 \text{ } \mu g}{1 \text{ ml}} = \begin{array}{c}\text{concentration}\\\text{of drip}\end{array}$$

Beginning the infusion at a rate of 2.5 μg/kg/min with an 80 kg patient, this would mean that 200 μg/min (2.5 × 80) must be infused.

If we wanted to infuse 1000 μg/min, the drip would have to be set at 60 drops/min (60 drops = 1 ml with a microdrip). Since we only want to infuse 200 μg/min, we have to set the drip at 12 drops/min (60 ÷ 5). (This drug does *not* obey the Rule of 250 ml.)

• • •

PROBLEM: Make up an infusion of sodium nitroprusside, and determine the speed of infusion needed to begin at a rate of 10 μg/min.

ANSWER: Mix 50 mg (1 vial) of nitroprusside in 250 ml of D_5W.

$$\frac{50 \text{ mg}}{250 \text{ ml}} = \frac{200 \text{ mg}}{1000 \text{ ml}} = \frac{200,000 \text{ } \mu g}{1000 \text{ ml}} = \frac{200 \text{ } \mu g}{\text{ml}} = \begin{array}{c}\text{concentration}\\\text{of drip}\end{array}$$

Beginning the infusion at 10 μg/min implies that $\frac{1}{20}$ ml/min must be infused.

Since 60 drops equal 1 ml with a microdrip, set the drip at 3 drops/min (60 ÷ 20) to begin the infusion rate at 10 μg/min.

PROBLEM: By how many drops per minute should the drip be increased to infuse an additional 10 μg each minute?

ANSWER: Since a rate of 3 drops/min infuses 10 μg/min, one would have to increase the drip by 3 drops each minute to infuse an additional 10 μg each minute.

PROBLEM: What is the maximum infusion rate recommended for an 80 kg patient?

ANSWER: The maximum recommended infusion rate is 8 μg/kg/min, which equals 80 × 8 or 640 μg/min.

At a concentration of 200 μg/ml, the maximum recommended infusion rate would be 3.2 ml/min, which equals 192 drops/min (60 × 3.2).

• • •

PROBLEM: Calculate an infusion of IV nitroglycerin.

ANSWER: Same method and doses as for sodium nitroprusside.

Mix 50 mg of nitroglycerin in 250 ml of D_5W, and set the drip to run at 3 drops/min to begin the infusion at 10 μg/min; increase the drip by 3 drops/min (10 μg/min) as needed to obtain the desired clinical response.

(Note that both sodium nitroprusside and nitroglycerin follow the Rule of 250 ml for preparing the concentration of infusion, but drips for these agents should be initally set at 3 drops/min (*not* 30 drops/min).

GUIDELINES FOR THE USE OF LIDOCAINE*

Lidocaine is the most commonly used antiarrhythmic agent for the emergency treatment of ventricular dysrhythmias. Despite its widespread use, opinions still vary about what constitutes the optimal protocol for administration of this drug. While virtually all therapeutic regimens employ an initial loading bolus, the need for one or more additional loading boluses remains open to question. Similarly, no general consensus exists regarding the ideal rate of infusion. Some authorities begin low (at an infusion rate of 1 mg/min) and adjust the infusion rate upward with each subsequent bolus, whereas others begin high (at an infusion rate of 4 mg/

*Figs. 3-2 to 3-8 are generated by SIMKIN software developed by J.D. Robinson at the University of Florida, College of Medicine and College of Pharmacy. SIMKIN software is operational on the IBM Personal Computer and the Hewlett-Packard 7470A Graphics Plotter.

min) and adjust the infusion rate downward. A third group maintains a constant infusion rate of 2 mg/min whether or not additional boluses of drug are given.

With such an abundance of treatment protocols to choose from it is not surprising that the emergency care provider often has difficulty deciding on the regimen best suited for a particular patient. This decision is further complicated by patient variables such as age, weight, the presence of acute myocardial infarction, congestive heart failure and/or liver disease, and the use of concomitant drugs, all of which may influence lidocaine metabolism. In an attempt to clarify the confusion surrounding the use of this drug, this chapter reviews the basic pharmacokinetic principles of lidocaine and illustrates how application of these principles allows one to optimize therapy and minimize the risk of toxicity. Finally, the issue of whether or not lidocaine should be given prophylactically to patients suspected of having acute myocardial infarction is discussed.

Lidocaine pharmacokinetics

Lidocaine pharmacokinetics can best be described by a two-compartment model (Fig. 3-1). The smaller *central compartment* includes the

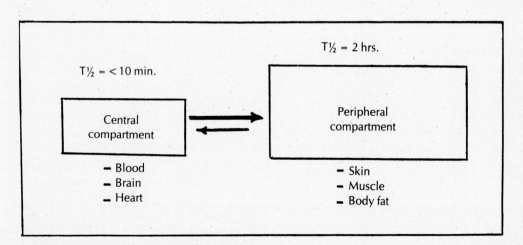

Fig. 3-1. Pharmacokinetic model for lidocaine.

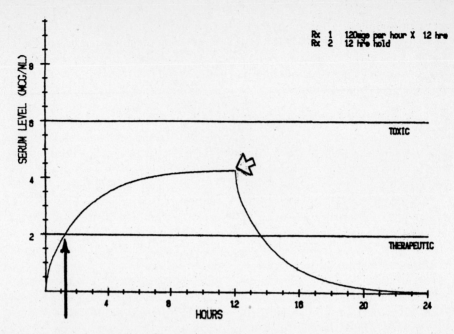

Fig. 3-2. A 50-year-old man (5 feet 10 inches, 75kg) with acute infarction is given an IV maintenance infusion of lidocaine at 2 mg/min. No loading dose is given. More than 1 hour passes before a therapeutic blood level is reached (arrow). The infusion is stopped after 12 hours (open arrowhead). Therapeutic blood levels persist for at least 2 hours.

circulating blood volume together with heart, brain, and other highly perfused organs. Because of redistribution into the peripheral compartment, the half-life of the drug in the central compartment is less than 10 minutes. The larger *peripheral compartment* includes poorly perfused tissues such as skin, muscle, and most of the body fat stores. In healthy adults the half-life of lidocaine in this space is usually 1 to 2 hours.

When a bolus of lidocaine is injected intravenously, it is administered directly into the central compartment. Since the heart is contained within this space, the antiarrhythmic effect of the drug begins almost immediately. Within 10 minutes, however, one half of the initial loading bolus is redistributed to the peripheral compartment, and the level of drug in the bloodstream drops significantly. PVCs may recur at this time

unless the serum drug concentration of lidocaine has been maintained within the therapeutic range (2 to 6 μg/ml) by additional loading boluses.

Lidocaine distribution from the central compartment to the peripheral compartment begins following an IV bolus and continues until a state of equilibrium is established between these two compartments. By administering one or more loading boluses, therapeutic blood levels are rapidly achieved and maintain an adequate antiarrhythmic effect until the continuous intravenous infusion has had an opportunity to attain steady state. If one were to simply institute a maintenance infusion without an initial loading dose, more than an hour would pass before serum drug levels would become therapeutic. This situation is illustrated in Fig. 3-2 in which a 75 kg man is given a maintenance infusion of 2 mg/min.

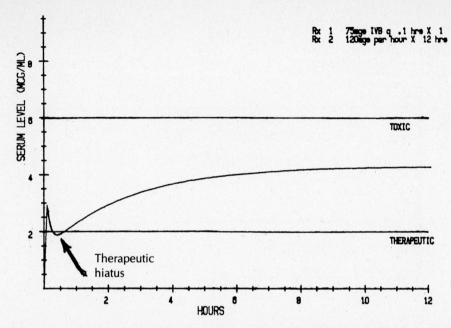

Fig. 3-3. The same man described in Fig 3-2 is initially given a 75 mg bolus of lidocaine before starting an IV maintenance infusion at 2 mg/min. Therapeutic blood levels are reached almost immediately. They then transiently dip into the subtherapeutic range (arrow) until steady state is established.

If the same 75 kg man is instead given a 75 mg loading bolus of lidocaine (1 mg/kg) before starting the 2 mg/min maintenance infusion, therapeutic drug levels of lidocaine would be reached almost immediately (Fig. 3-3). With the exception of a momentary dip below the therapeutic range (arrow in Fig. 3-3), adequate blood levels are maintained until steady state is established. If one were to follow the initial 75 mg loading bolus with a second bolus given a short time later, even this transient "therapeutic hiatus" might be avoided (Fig. 3-4).

The eventual steady state serum drug level (which in this case is just over 4 μg/ml) might be reached even sooner if a third and/or fourth loading bolus were administered (Fig. 3-5). This type of aggressive loading protocol calls for an initial loading dose of 75 mg followed by 50 mg boluses every 5 minutes until a total loading

dose of up to 225 mg has been given. One may either keep the infusion rate constant at 2 mg/min (as in Fig. 3-5) or increase the infusion rate by 1 mg/min after each additional loading bolus is given until a maximum rate of 4 mg/min is reached. The problem is that even in an otherwise healthy 50-year-old man, the presence of any complicating factors that retard lidocaine metabolism (acute infarction, shock, congestive failure, or concomitant use of drugs such as propranolol or cimetidine) may be enough to cause the patient to become toxic when higher infusion rates are used (Fig. 3-6).

Actually one should not have to increase the rate of infusion even if breakthrough PVCs occur during the initial hour of the loading period. The reason PVCs might recur 10 to 20 minutes following the loading bolus in Fig. 3-3 is not because the rate of the maintenance infusion is

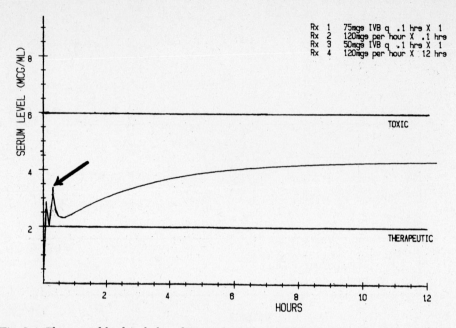

Fig. 3-4. The second loading bolus of 50 mg (arrow) is given 5 minutes after the initial 75 mg loading dose. Blood levels never drop into the subtherapeutic range.

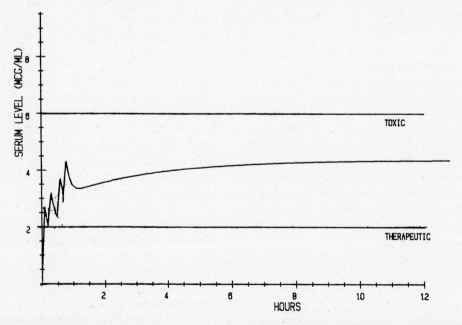

Fig. 3-5. Loading regimen whereby the same man shown previously is given an initial loading dose of 75 mg followed by three additional 50 mg boluses spaced 5 minutes apart. The maintenance infusion is set at 2 mg/min.

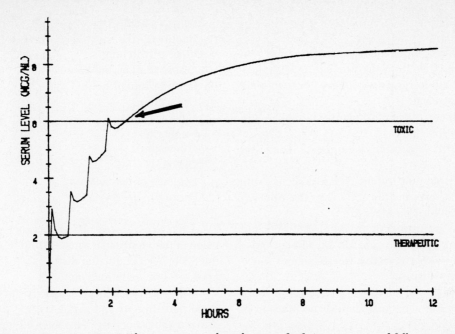

Fig. 3-6. Patient in Fig. 3-5 becomes toxic when the rate of infusion is increased following each loading dose (arrow).

too slow but rather because of the drop in the level of lidocaine in the blood as the drug is redistributed from the central compartment to the peripheral compartment. This drop could be avoided by administering one or more additional loading boluses (Figs. 3-4 and 3-5). The eventual steady state plasma concentration of lidocaine is *not* influenced by the manner in which the patient is loaded. As long as the rate of the maintenance infusion remains constant at 2 mg/min, the eventual level of lidocaine in the blood will be the same (a steady state level of just over 4 μg/ml is ultimately reached in Figs. 3-3 to 3-5). Only if a serum drug level of greater than 4 μg/ml is required for dysrhythmia control would one have to increase the rate of the maintenance infusion above 2 mg/min.

In summary, a reasonable protocol for administering lidocaine is to initially give the patient a 50 to 100 mg IV bolus (1 mg/kg) and to simulta-

neously start a maintenance infusion at 2 mg/min. If lidocaine is being used purely as a prophylactic measure to prevent ventricular fibrillation in a patient suspected of acute infarction but without ventricular ectopy, additional loading boluses would not be needed (Fig. 3-3). Alternatively, one might administer a second loading bolus of 50 to 75 mg 5 to 10 minutes after the initial bolus (Fig. 3-4). More aggressive loading (Fig. 3-5) only increases the risk of toxicity and probably is not warranted when using lidocaine prophylactically.

On the other hand, when lidocaine is being used to treat frequent and complex ventricular ectopy, one may choose to follow the initial loading dose with one or more additional 50 to 75 mg boluses spaced 5 to 10 minutes apart until a total loading dose of up to 225 mg has been given. If ventricular ectopy is controlled as this regimen is administered, the rate of the maintenance infusion need not necessarily be increased after each bolus.

A number of questions on the usage of lidocaine may arise from the preceding discussion:

- Why are loading doses of greater than 1 mg/kg not used?
- What are the clinical manifestations of lidocaine toxicity?
- How is lidocaine eliminated from the body?
- When administration of lidocaine is being halted, can one abruptly stop the infusion, or should it be tapered?
- What adjustments in administering lidocaine should be made for the elderly and/or those with congestive heart failure, shock, or liver disease?
- When should lidocaine be used prophylactically? For how long should the infusion be maintained?

Optimal loading dose of lidocaine

The optimal initial loading dose of lidocaine is a 1 mg/kg bolus given intravenously. Despite common usage of the term *bolus*, this dose should be infused over a 1 to 2 minute period so as not to flood the central compartment with the drug. As mentioned previously, since the heart is contained within the central space, the antiarrhythmic effect of a loading dose begins almost immediately. The brain is also contained within this central compartment, however, and too rapid infusion of the loading bolus or too large a dose may produce central nervous system toxicity. Thus although doses of greater than 1 mg/kg of lidocaine might be more effective in obtaining the necessary level of the drug in the patient, they are not recommended because of the unwarranted risk of toxicity.

Manifestations of toxicity

The clinical manifestations of lidocaine toxicity principally involve the central nervous system and include the following:

Increasing blood level ↑
- Respiratory arrest
- Seizures
- Muscle twitching
- Disorientation and confusion
- Hearing impairment
- Dysarthria
- Mild agitation
- Euphoria
- Drowsiness
- Dizziness
- Feelings of dissociation
- Perioral paresthesias

Adverse cardiovascular effects such as depression of left ventricular function and exacerbation of SA or AV conduction disturbances may occur but are distinctly uncommon.

Mild signs of lidocaine toxicity such as perioral paresthesias and dizziness may be seen at serum drug concentrations near 5 μg/ml, a level that overlaps with the upper limits of the therapeutic range. These adverse reactions commonly follow infusion of a loading bolus, especially if the drug is administered too rapidly. In this case there should be prompt resolution of such side effects. If similar adverse reactions occur during a maintenance infusion, however, they should be taken as evidence of drug accumulation and impending toxicity. The drip should be immediately stopped and blood should be drawn to determine drug level.

The problem with diagnosing lidocaine toxicity is that severe reactions such as seizures and respiratory arrest may occasionally occur without the milder premonitory symptoms. A patient convulsing during cardiac arrest may be hypoxic, hypotensive, alkalotic, or toxic from lidocaine. Since clinical assessment without laboratory confirmation has not been shown to be accurate in differentiating among these possibilities (Deglin et al., 1980), cautious dosing and a high index of suspicion are advised when treating patients at high risk of developing toxicity.

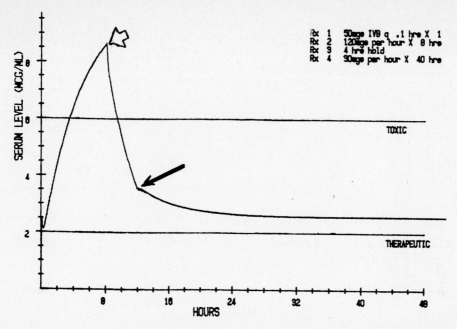

Fig. 3-7. A 70-year-old woman (5 feet 2 inches, 50 kg) with acute infarction and pulmonary edema is given a 50 mg bolus and a maintenance infusion of 2 mg/min. The infusion is held after 8 hours (open arrowhead) when she becomes toxic, and then it is restarted at 12 hours (arrow) at the lower infusion rate of ½ mg/min.

Lidocaine elimination and adjustments in dosing

Lidocaine is eliminated from the body by hepatic metabolism. The half-life of this elimination phase is proportional to hepatic blood flow, and under normal circumstances it takes between 1 and 2 hours. Patients in shock or congestive heart failure in whom hepatic blood flow may be greatly diminished would be expected to have a prolonged elimination phase half-life and be more susceptible to accumulation of drug and lidocaine toxicity. Other groups at high risk of developing lidocaine toxicity include patients with liver disease, those taking drugs such as propranolol or cimetidine that decrease hepatic clearance of lidocaine, the elderly in whom cardiac output is less, and patients with low body weight. In addition, the elimination phase half-life of lidocaine may increase in patients with

acute infarction or in those taking prolonged (≥ 24 hour) infusions of the drug. For this reason one often decreases the rate of the maintenance infusion in patients on lidocaine for more than 24 hours.

Abruptly stopping an IV maintenance infusion of lidocaine will *not* immediately result in subtherapeutic blood levels. This point is well illustrated by Fig. 3-2, in which serum drug levels do not fall into the subtherapeutic range for nearly 2 hours after the maintenance infusion is discontinued. Thus there would seem to be no rationale for tapering patients off lidocaine infusions, since the 1- to 2-hour elimination phase half-life of the drug automatically ensures a tapering effect.

What adjustments in dosing should be made for those patients at high risk of developing lidocaine toxicity? Consider the case of the 50 kg

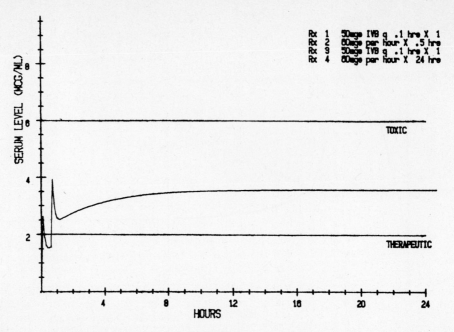

Fig. 3-8. A 70-year-old woman (5 feet 2 inches, 50 kg) with acute infarction but without congestive heart failure is given two 50 mg loading boluses and then is maintained on an IV infusion at 1 mg/min.

elderly woman (shown in Fig. 3-7) who is admitted with pulmonary edema from an acute myocardial infarction. After receiving the standard 1 mg/kg loading dose (in this case 50 mg), she rapidly became toxic on a maintenance infusion rate of 2 mg/min. This rate is too high for an elderly patient of low body weight with acute infarction and significant congestive heart failure. After holding the infusion for 4 hours (open arrowhead), the drip was restarted (arrow) at a new infusion rate of ½ mg/min. In a patient such as this an infusion rate of ½ mg/min may be adequate to maintain a therapeutic drug level.

Let us assume that this same 50 kg elderly woman was admitted with an acute myocardial infarction but without any signs of congestive heart failure. In this case one might achieve and maintain therapeutic blood levels by administering two 50 mg loading boluses and running a constant IV infusion at 1 mg/min (Fig. 3-8).

In summary, it is important to lower the rate of the lidocaine maintenance infusion in the elderly, in patients with low body weight, and/or those with complicating factors such as congestive heart failure or shock.

Prophylactic use of lidocaine

In the past it was thought that "warning arrhythmias" (five or more PVCs per minute, two or more PVCs in a row, multifocal PVCs, the "R-on-T" phenomenon) regularly preceded the development of primary ventricular fibrillation in patients with acute myocardial infarction. Consequently, one would wait for the occurrence of such arrhythmias before initiating antiarrhythmic treatment in patients admitted with acute chest pain.

Today the concept of warning arrhythmias has been conclusively disproven. Ventricular fibrillation frequently occurs in acute myocardial infarction without warning arrhythmias. Sometimes it even occurs without any prior ectopic activity. Moreover, when warning arrhythmias do occur, they do not reliably predict which patients will subsequently develop ventricular fibrillation.

In view of the fact that 5% to 10% of all patients with acute myocardial infarction develop primary ventricular fibrillation, it would seem prudent to consider the prophylactic use of antiarrhythmic therapy. Lidocaine has been the drug most commonly chosen for this purpose. It is easy to administer, is well tolerated by most patients, and effectively lowers the incidence of primary ventricular fibrillation associated with acute infarction. This drug should not be used indiscriminately, however, since its administration is associated with a 5% to 15% incidence of toxicity. The risk of lidocaine toxicity seems to be greatest for patients over 70 years old (Goldman et al., 1979; Lie et al., 1974). Since the risk of developing primary ventricular fibrillation is significantly less in this age group, elderly patients could reasonably be excluded from consideration for lidocaine prophylaxis.

Patients most likely to benefit from lidocaine prophylaxis are those seen early during the course of their illness and in whom a high index of suspicion for acute infarction exists. This is because the greatest incidence of primary ventricular fibrillation associated with acute myocardial infarction occurs within the first few hours of the onset of symptoms. It is rare after 24 hours, and lidocaine prophylaxis is probably not warranted in patients who are first seen after this period.

It is important to differentiate primary ventricular fibrillation from the secondary form of ventricular fibrillation. This latter condition characteristically occurs several days after the onset of symptoms and is associated with the development of cardiogenic shock. As one might expect, the secondary form of ventricular fibrillation is notoriously resistant to any type of antiarrhythmic therapy.

In summary, the prophylactic use of lidocaine for the prevention of primary ventricular fibrillation associated with acute myocardial infarction is probably reasonable in the following cases:

- Patients under 70 years of age
- Those seen within the first 24 hours of the onset of symptoms
- Those in whom a high index of suspicion for acute infarction exists

These patients should be given one or two IV loading boluses of lidocaine, and a continuous infusion of 1 to 2 mg/min should be started regardless of whether or not they are manifesting ventricular ectopic activity.

SUGGESTED READINGS

Adgey, A.A.J., Geddes, J.S., Webb, S.W., Allen, J.D., James, R.G.G., Zaidi, S.A., and Pantridge, J.F.: Acute phase of myocardial infarction, Lancet 2:501-504, 1971.

Barnaby, P.F., Barrett, P.A., and Lvoff, R.: Routine prophylactic lidocaine in acute myocardial infarction, Heart Lung 12:362-366, 1983.

Church, G., and Biern, R.O.: Intensive coronary care—a practical system for a small hospital without house staff, N. Engl. J. Med. 281:1155-1159, 1969.

Deglin, S.M., Deglin, J.M., Wurtzbacher, J., Litton, M., Rolfe, C., and McIntire, C.: Rapid serum lidocaine determination in the coronary care unit, JAMA 244:571-573, 1980.

El-Sherif, N., Myerberg, R.J., Scherlag, B.J., Befeler, B., Aranda, J.M., Castellanos, A., and Lazzara, R.: Electrocardiographic antecedents of primary ventricular fibrillation, Br. Heart J. 38:415-422, 1976.

Fuchs, R., and Scheidt, S.: Improved criteria for admission to cardiac care units, JAMA 246:2037-2041, 1981.

Goldman, L., and Batsford, W.F.: Risk-benefit stratification as a guide to lidocaine prophylaxis of primary ventricular fibrillation in acute myocardial infarction: an analytic review, Yale J. Biol. Med. 52:455-466, 1979.

Grauer, K.: Should prophylactic lidocaine be routinely used in patients suspected of acute myocardial infarction? J. Fla. Med. Assoc. 69:377-379, 1982.

Harrison, D.: Should lidocaine be administered routinely to all patients after acute myocardial infarction? Circulation 58:581-584, 1978.

Lie, K.I., Wellens, H.J., van Capelle, F.J., and Durrer, D.: Lidocaine in prevention of primary ventricular fibrillation, New Engl. J. Med. 291:1324-1326, 1974.

Meltzer, L.F., and Kitchell, J.R.: Incidence of arrhythmias associated with acute myocardial infarction, Prog. Cardiovasc. Dis. 9:50-63, 1966.

Romhilt, D.W., Boomfield, S.S., Chou, T.C., and Fowler, N.O.: Unreliability of conventional electrocardiographic monitoring for arrhythmia detection in coronary care units, Am. J. Cardiol. 31:457-461, 1973.

Seager, S.B.: Cardiac enzymes in evaluation of chest pain, Ann. Emerg. Med. 9:346-349, 1980.

Sobel, B.E., and Braunwald, E.: Management of acute myocardial infarction. In Braunwald, E.: Heart disease, Philadelphia, 1980, W.B. Saunders Co., pp. 1360-1363.

Stargel, W.W., and Routledge, P.A.: Lidocaine: therapeutic use and serum concentration monitoring. In Taylor, W.J., and Finn, A.L., editor: Individualizing drug therapy, New York, 1981, Gross, Townsend, Frank, Inc., pp. 1-21.

Wyman, M.G., and Hammersmith, L.: Comprehensive treatment plan for prevention of primary ventricular fibrillation in acute myocardial infarction, Am. J. Cardiol. 33:661-667, 1974.

Wyman, M.G., and Goldreyer, B.N.: No arrhythmia deaths in 1000 acute myocardial infarctions (abstract), Circulation 53-54(suppl. 2):524, 1976.

Wyman, M.G., and Gore, S.: Lidocaine prophylaxis in myocardial infarction: a concept whose time has come, Heart Lung 12:358-361, 1983.

PART TWO

DYSRHYTHMIA RECOGNITION

CHAPTER 4

Rate and rhythm

Although the ability to rapidly and accurately determine *rate* and *rhythm* is a prerequisite skill for successfully managing cardiac arrest, it remains an obstacle to many of those who do not deal with acute cardiac emergencies on a daily basis. The goal of this chapter is to explore some of the dysrhythmias that are usually encountered during the course of cardiac resuscitation and to offer a readily mastered approach to interpretation.

RATE

Heart rate may be calculated at a glance. At the standard speed of recording (25 mm/sec.), the amount of time required to travel the distance represented by one *large box* on ECG paper is 0.20 second. If a QRS complex were to occur every large box (every 0.20 second), five QRS complexes would occur in 1 second (0.20 second × 5 = 1.0 second). Since there are 60 seconds in a minute, the heart rate would be 300 beats/min. (5 beats/sec × 60 sec/min = 300 beats/min).

PROBLEM: Examine Fig. 4-1 taken from a patient who has just become pulseless and unresponsive. What is the rhythm? What is the rate of this rhythm?

ANSWER TO FIG. 4-1: Clinically one would expect to find ventricular fibrillation in a patient who has just become pulseless and unresponsive. Instead, a rapid and regularly occurring complex appears on the monitor. This complex occurs every large box, making its rate about 300 beats/min. Since this is too rapid a ventricular response for virtually any dysrhythmia in an adult, the rhythm is most likely artifactual. (One of the monitoring leads had become disconnected, accounting for the artifact. When reapplied, the patient was found to be in ventricular fibrillation.)

• • •

PROBLEM: Unlike the ventricles, the atria may contract 300 times/min. The patient in Fig. 4-2 is in atrial flutter. A flutter wave occurs in about one large box of time, making the atrial rate approximately 300 beats/min (small arrowheads). How many flutter waves are there for each QRS complex? How fast is the ventricular rate in Fig. 4-2?

ANSWER TO FIG. 4-2: The interval between each QRS complex (the R-R interval) in Fig. 4-2 is about four large boxes (large arrowheads). Since the heart rate of a patient having a QRS complex each large box would be 300 beats/min, the heart rate should be one fourth as much if a QRS complex occurs every four boxes (300 ÷ 4 = 75 beats/min). There are four atrial flutter waves for each QRS complex (there is 4:1 AV conduction). (If you are hav-

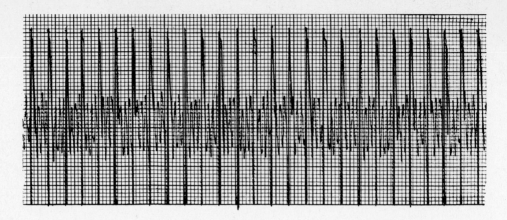

Fig. 4-1

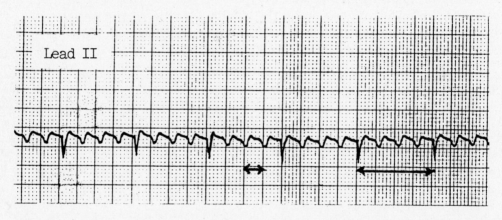

Fig. 4-2. From Grauer, K., and Curry, R.W., Jr.: Monograph 47, AAFP Home Study Self-Assessment, © 1983, American Academy of Family Physicians.

ing trouble spotting the fourth flutter wave, it is buried in the QRS complex.)

A rapid and accurate method of estimating heart rate is to *divide 300 by the number of boxes that make up the R-R interval (Fig. 4-3).* If a QRS complex occurs every two large boxes, the heart rate is $300 \div 2 = 150$ beats/min; a QRS every three large boxes reflects a heart rate of $300 \div 3 = 100$ beats/min; a QRS every four large boxes reflects a rate of 75 beats/min and so on.

• • •

PROBLEM: What is the approximate rate of the SVT shown in Fig. 4-4?

ANSWER TO FIG. 4-4: The R-R interval in Fig. 4-4 appears to be just under two large boxes in duration. (The easiest way to estimate this without calipers is to locate a QRS complex that begins on one of the heavy lines as indicated by the arrow, and then to count over to the next QRS complex.) If the R-R interval were exactly two large boxes, then the rate would be 150 beats/min ($300 \div 2$). Since it is

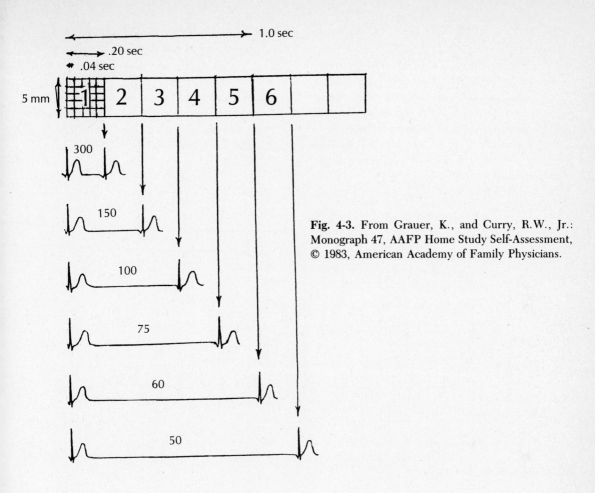

Fig. 4-3. From Grauer, K., and Curry, R.W., Jr.: Monograph 47, AAFP Home Study Self-Assessment, © 1983, American Academy of Family Physicians.

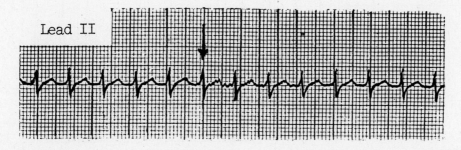

Fig. 4-4. From Grauer, K., and Curry, R.W., Jr.: Monograph 47, AAFP Home Study Self-Assessment, © 1983, American Academy of Family Physicians.

less than two boxes, the rate is between 150 and 300 beats/min and closer to the former.

When the rate is extremely rapid (between 150 and 300 beats/min), accurate estimation of heart rate becomes difficult, since minor discrepancies in how one measures the R-R interval may make a fairly large difference in the calculated rate. For example, it is hard to be sure if the rate in Fig. 4-4 is above or below 200 beats/min.

A handy trick to use when the rate is fast and regular is to measure the R-R interval of two beats (or of one half the actual rate). In Fig. 4-4 the R-R interval of two beats is about 3½ boxes. Thus *one half the acutal rate* is nearly midway between 100 and 75 beats/min (between three and four large boxes, respectively), or about 85 to 90 beats/min. The actual rate is therefore about 175 beats/min (87.5 × 2.0)

• • •

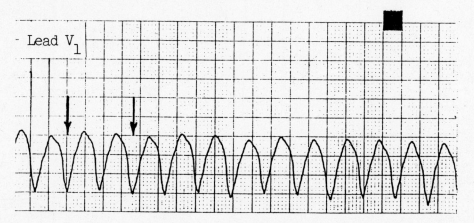

Fig. 4-5. From Grauer, K., and Curry, R.W., Jr.: Monograph 47, AAFP Home Study Self-Assessment, © 1983, American Academy of Family Physicians.

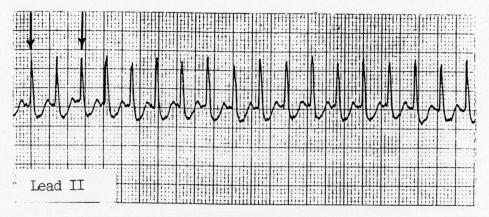

Fig. 4-6. From Grauer, K., and Curry, R.W., Jr.: Monograph 47, AAFP Home Study Self-Assessment, © 1983, American Academy of Family Physicians.

PROBLEM: Try this technique on the examples shown in Fig. 4-5 and 4-6. Is the rate of one or both of these rhythms over 200 beats/min?

ANSWER TO FIG. 4-5: The arrows in Fig. 4-5 show the R-R interval for *two* beats to be between three and four boxes and closer to the latter. Thus *half* the actual rate is 80 beats/min; the actual rate is about 160 beats/min.

ANSWER TO FIG. 4-6: The arrows indicate that the R-R interval for *two* beats in Fig. 4-6 is between two and three boxes and much closer to the latter. Thus *half* the actual rate is between 150 and 100 beats/min and probably about 110 beats/min. The actual rate is therefore 220 beats/min (110 × 2).

The QRS complex in Fig. 4-5 is wide (at least 0.16 second), although it is hard to determine where the QRS complex ends and the ST segment begins. No P waves are seen. One must assume that this is *ventricular tachycardia* until proven otherwise.

• • •

PROBLEM: Can you think of two other diagnostic possibilities for the rhythm shown in Fig. 4-5?

ANSWER: One cannot absolutely rule out SVT with either preexisting bundle branch block or aberrant conduction on the basis of the tracing in Fig. 4-5 alone.

In Fig. 4-6 the QRS complex appears to be narrow (≤ 0.10 second). Although there is no way to tell if P waves are hidden within the ST segment, definite atrial activity cannot be identified. This rhythm could be paroxysmal atrial tachycardia (PAT) or paroxysmal junctional tachycardia (PJT). Differentiation between these two entities is often impossible, and this difficulty is acknowledged by the rhythm being called *paroxysmal supraventricular tachycardia (PSVT)*.

• • •

PROBLEM: Could the rhythm in Fig. 4-6 also be atrial flutter? Could it be sinus tachycardia?

ANSWER: The atrial rate in flutter most often hovers around 300 beats/min (range 250 to 350) except when it has been slowed by a medication such as quinidine. The AV node is unable to conduct each atrial impulse at this rapid rate, which is fortunate, since effective cardiac pumping could not be maintained at 300 beats/min. However, the AV node *is* able to conduct every other atrial impulse. Thus *the most common ventricular response in untreated atrial flutter is 2:1* (an atrial rate of 300 beats/min and *a ventricular response of 150 beats/min*). Less often there is 4:1 AV conduction (as in Fig. 4-2) or variable AV conduction.

The ventricular rate in Fig. 4-6 is much faster than the usual 150 beats/min that would normally be expected in atrial flutter, making this diagnosis unlikely. Similarily, it would be unusual for sinus tachycardia to be faster than 150 to 160 beats/min in an adult. This leaves PSVT as the most probable diagnosis.

• • •

PROBLEM: Estimate the rate of the slow rhythms shown in Figs. 4-7 to 4-9. From where in the conduction system would you expect these rhythms to arise?

ANSWER TO FIG. 4-7: The R-R interval of the rhythm in Fig. 4-7 is a little over six boxes. The rate is therefore just under 50 beats/min. No P waves are seen, and the QRS complex is wide, making this an accelerated idioventricular rhythm (AIVR). (It is an "escape rhythm" because the sinus pacemaker has failed, and it is "accelerated" because the usual rate of an idioventricular rhythm is 30 to 40 beats/min.)

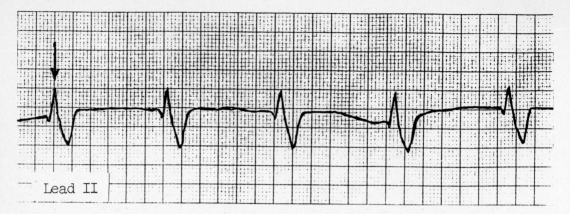

Lead II

Fig. 4-7. From Grauer, K., and Curry, R.W., Jr.: Monograph 47, AAFP Home Study Self-Assessment, © 1983, American Academy of Family Physicians.

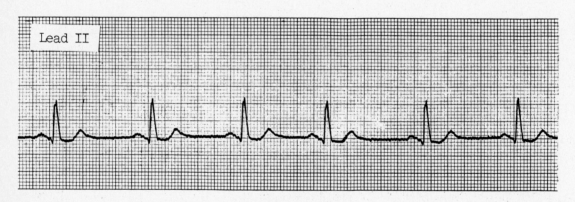

Lead II

Fig. 4-8

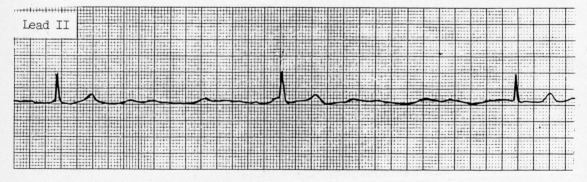

Lead II

Fig. 4-9. From Grauer, K., and Curry, R.W., Jr.: Monograph 47, AAFP Home Study Self-Assessment, © 1983, American Academy of Family Physicians.

ANSWER TO FIG. 4-8: The R-R interval of the rhythm in Fig. 4-8 is slightly irregular and averages out to between five and six boxes. Thus the rate is between 50 and 60 beats/min. Close inspection of the QRS complex reveals it to be wide; it is almost three little boxes in duration (0.11 to 0.12 second). Yet unlike the rhythm in Fig. 4-7, each QRS complex is preceded by a normal-appearing P wave with a constant PR interval. Clearly a sinus mechanism is operative here. *Sinus bradycardia* is present, since the rate is under 60 beats/min, and there is *sinus arrhythmia*, since the R-R interval varies. The QRS prolongation can be explained by the existence of an intraventricular conduction delay.

ANSWER TO FIG. 4-9: The R-R interval of the rhythm in Fig. 4-9 is almost 15 boxes, corresponding to a rate of about 20 beats/min (300 ÷ 15). Despite this slow rate, the QRS complex is narrow. This makes the rhythm less likely to arise from a ventricular focus. Sinus mechanism is precluded by the fact that P waves are absent. Thus Fig. 4-9 probably represents an escape rhythm that arises from low down in the conduction system (from the His or the bundle branches).

Without specifically addressing this issue, we have already alluded to the *principal determinants of rhythm*, which include the following:
- Rate
- Regularity (or the lack of it)
- Presence (or absence) of P waves
- Relationship of P waves to the QRS complex
- Width of the QRS complex

Attention to these five factors explains most basic dysrhythmias.

• • •

PROBLEM: Concentrate on the presence of P waves and their meaning. Examine the rhythms shown in Figs. 4-10 to 4-13. What is the mechanism of each of these dysrhythmias? Are P waves present? Are they related to the QRS complex?

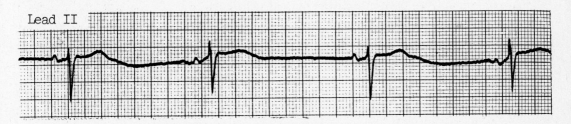

Fig. 4-10

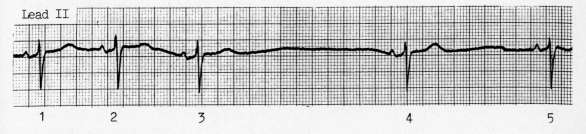

Fig. 4-11

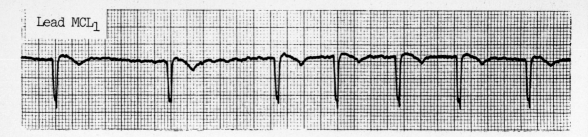

Lead MCL₁

Fig. 4-12

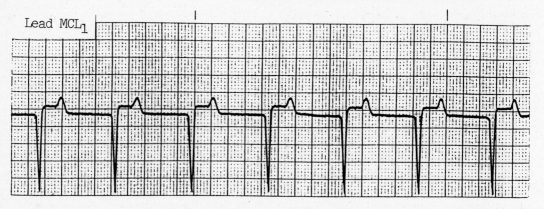

Lead MCL₁

Fig. 4-13. From Grauer, K., and Curry, R.W., Jr.: Monograph 47, AAFP Home Study Self-Assessment, © 1983, American Academy of Family Physicians.

ANSWER TO FIG. 4-10: In Fig. 4-10 a slow, slightly irregular rhythm is present with a heart rate of about 35 beats/min (the R-R interval is between 8 and 9 boxes; $300 \div 8.5 \approx 35$). The QRS complex is narrow, and a P wave with a constant PR interval precedes each QRS complex, indicating sinus mechanism. Like Fig. 4-8, this is *sinus bradycardia* and *sinus arrhythmia*.

ANSWER TO FIG. 4-11: The tracing in Fig. 4-11 is taken from the same patient as was Fig. 4-10. Sinus rhythm at a rate of about 60 beats/min is manifest for the first three beats, after which long pauses precede the next two QRS complexes. However, the QRS configuration of beats 4 and 5 is identical to that of the first three beats, and sinus P waves with a constant

PR interval precede all five QRS complexes in the rhythm strip. Thus the basic rhythm is *sinus* with *sinus pauses* following beats 3 and 4. The combination of sinus arrhythmia, bradycardia, and sinus pauses seen in Figs. 4-10 and 4-11 suggests that the patient has *sick sinus syndrome*.

ANSWER TO FIG. 4-12: In Fig 4-12 the rhythm is *irregularly irregular* (the R-R intervals continuously vary). No P waves are evident anywhere. This is *atrial fibrillation* by definition.

ANSWER TO FIG. 4-13: The rhythm is fairly regular at a rate of about 65 beats/min in Fig. 4-13. Again no P waves are evident, but the regularity of the rhythm and the normal dura-

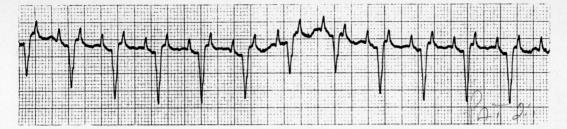

Fig. 4-14

tion of the QRS complex suggest that this is a *junctional rhythm*.

The last four examples (Figs. 4-14 to 4-17) test your mettle. Although analysis of these dysrhythmias is somewhat involved, application of the principles discussed and summarized in this chapter (box opposite) should make possible the identification of P waves, the determination of their relation to the QRS complex, the assessment of the regularity of rhythm and the width of the QRS complex, and the estimation of the atrial and ventricular rates. Extension of these principles to the various dysrhythmias encountered during cardiac arrest should facilitate rapid and accurate interpretation.

ANSWER TO FIG. 4-14: In Fig. 4-14 the rhythm is regular with a ventricular rate of about 115 beats/min (the R-R interval is between two and three boxes and closer to the latter). P waves outnumber QRS complexes by two to one, making the atrial rate about 230 beats/min. The QRS complex is narrow, implying a supraventricular mechanism, and each QRS complex is preceded by a P wave with a constant PR interval. Thus P waves *are* related to the QRS complexes, albeit only one out of every two P waves is conducted to the ventricles. This is *PAT with 2:1 AV block,* a rhythm that is frequently associated with digitalis toxicity.

● ● ●

PRACTICAL APPROACH TO DYSRHYTH-MIA INTERPRETATION

1. Are P waves present?
2. Is the rhythm regular?
   a. Regularity of R-R interval?
   b. Regularity of P-P interval?
3. What is the heart rate?
   a. Atrial rate?
   b. Ventricular rate?
   c. Too irregular to tell?
4. Is the QRS complex wide or narrow?
5. Are the P waves related to the QRS complex?
   a. Each QRS complex preceded by a P wave?
   b. PR interval normal?
   c. More P waves than QRS complexes?

PROBLEM: Why could Fig. 4-14 not also represent atrial flutter with 2:1 AV conduction?

ANSWER: Fig. 4-14 could also represent atrial flutter with 2:1 AV conduction. However, the atrial rate in flutter most often is close to 300 beats/min. Thus the slower atrial rate present in this example is less likely to be flutter unless the patient is taking a medication such as quinidine that slows the atrial rate. Another factor favoring PAT with block is that the baseline between P waves is flat (isoelectric). The sawtooth pattern commonly seen with flutter is absent here.

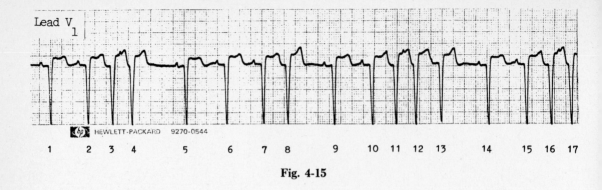

Lead V₁

Fig. 4-15

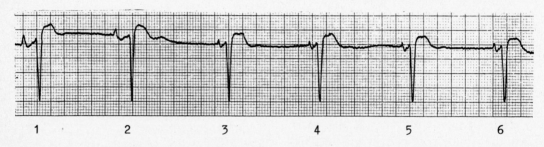

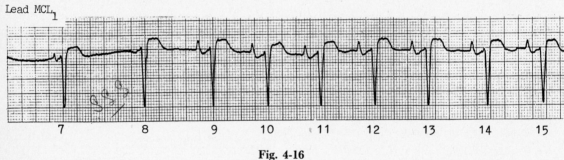

Lead MCL₁

Fig. 4-16

ANSWER TO FIG. 4-15: The rhythm in Fig. 4-15 is irregularly irregular, but atrial fibrillation is not present because P waves precede many of the QRS complexes. The QRS complex itself is narrow, and similar-appearing P waves with a constant PR interval precede beats 1, 2, 5, 6, 7, 9, 10, 14, and 15. Inspection of the T waves preceding beats 4, 11, 12, 16, and 17 reveals a notching that differentiates these T waves from normal T-wave morphology. (Normal T waves follow beats 1, 5, 6, 9, and 14). This notching is the result of the presence of premature P waves, making beats 4, 11, 12, 16, and 17 PACs. Beats 3 and 8 occur early, but there is no obvious deformity of the T wave preceding them. They are probably premature junctional contractions (PJCs). Thus the basic rhythm for Fig 4-15 is *sinus* with *frequent PACs* and *PJCs*.

ANSWER TO FIG. 4-16: P waves are readily identifiable in Fig. 14-16, but their morphology

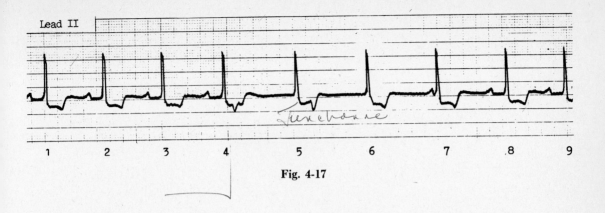

Fig. 4-17

changes. The first two complexes (beats 1 and 2) are preceded by a peaked P wave and are conducted with first-degree AV block (PR interval >0.20 second). The P wave morphology then changes and takes on a biphasic configuration for beats 3 to 7, all of which are conducted with a normal PR interval. A negative P wave precedes beat 8 followed by resumption of the peaked P-wave configuration and acceleration of the rate. This figure illustrates a *wandering atrial pacemaker, sinus bradycardia*, and *sinus arrhythmia*, all components of the *SSS*.

ANSWER TO FIG. 4-17: In Fig. 4-17 the first four beats are sinus conducted with first-degree AV block. The rate slows down beginning with beat 5. A supraventricular mechanism is maintained throughout, since the QRS remains narrow. However, whereas P waves consistently precede beats 1 to 4 with a con-

stant PR interval, no such P waves precede beats 5 and 6. These are junctional beats. (One wonders whether the negative notching in the T waves following beats 4 and 5 are retrograde P waves.) A normal-appearing P wave again precedes beat 7 but with a PR interval that is much too short to conduct. Thus this P wave is *not* related to QRS complex 7 (i.e., it is "dissociated" from it). Acceleration of the rate and return to sinus rhythm occurs by beat 9. Fig. 17 therefore illustrates an *underlying sinus rhythm* with *transient AV dissociation* and an appropriate junctional escape rhythm.

SUGGESTED READING

Grauer, K, and Curry, R.W.: Interpreting ECGs: a workbook (monograph 47), Kansas City, Mo., 1983, American Academy of Family Physicians Home Study Self-Assessment.

CHAPTER 5

Differentiation of PVCs from aberrancy

One of the most difficult problems confronting those involved in emergency cardiac care is the differentiation of PVCs from aberrantly conducted beats. The issue is not merely academic. Whereas ventricular dysrhythmias may be potentially life-threatening if not adequately controlled, supraventricular beats that conduct aberrantly are most often benign and can usually be safely observed without treatment.

PROBLEM: How can one reliably distinguish between PVCs and aberrancy? Can one always be sure of this differentiation? For example, examine the rhythm strips of the two patients on telemetry shown in Figs. 5-1 and 5-2. Should one of these patients be treated for ventricular ectopy? Should both be treated?

The purpose of this chapter is to furnish some guidelines with which one should be able to answer these questions *most* of the time. It is important to emphasize that occasionally it may be impossible to differentiate between PVCs and aberrantly conducted beats. In these cases correlation of the dysrhythmia to the clinical situation becomes critical. For example, the treatment of choice for a hemodynamically significant tachydysrhythmia is cardioversion regardless of whether the dysrhythmia is superventricular or ventricular in nature.

The burden of proof should lie with demonstrating that an abnormal-appearing QRS complex is aberrant rather than the other way around. Thus "a beat should be judged guilty (a PVC) until proven innocent!" Application of the basic principles presented in this chapter (and use of a pair of calipers) should increase the reader's confidence in making this judgment. (The two examples presented in Figs. 5-1 and 5-2 are discussed later in this chapter.)

BASIC RULES FOR DIFFERENTIATING PVCS FROM ABERRANCY

Three of the most helpful characteristics of aberrantly conducted beats are the following:
- *RBBB* pattern in a right-sided monitoring lead (lead V_1 or MCL_1)
- *Similar initial deflection* of the anomalous and normally conducted beats
- *Premature* P wave.

These features are well illustrated in the aberrantly conducted complex shown in Fig. 5-3. Although beat 4 in this rhythm strip looks markedly different from the others, it manifests an RBBB pattern (an rSR′ in a right-sided lead), and its initial QRS deflection is in the same direction as for the normally conducted beats (upward). Careful inspection of the T wave immediately preceding beat 4 reveals some extra peaking compared to the normal T waves.

64

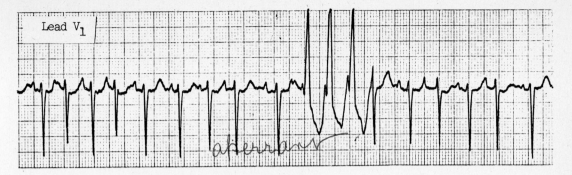

Lead V_1

Fig. 5-1

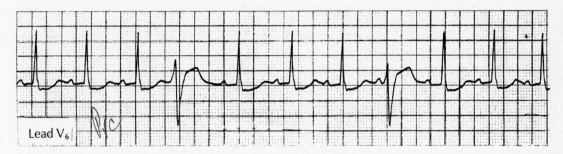

Lead V_6

Fig. 5-2

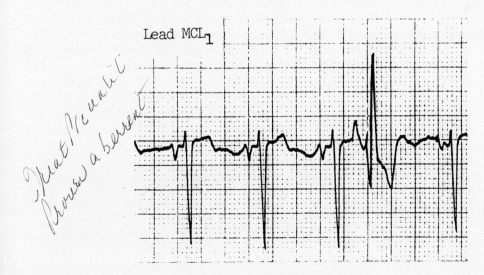

Lead MCL_1

Fig. 5-3

This is because of a premature P wave.

The reason aberrant beats frequently conduct with an RBBB pattern is that the refractory period of the right bundle branch tends to be longer than that of the left bundle branch. Thus it is common for a premature impulse arriving at the ventricles to find the right bundle branch still in a refractory state.

The initial deflection of aberrant beats is usually similar to that of the normally conducted beats, since the initial portion of the conduction pathway is usually unaffected; the wave of depolarization is conducted normally until it encounters that part of the conduction system that is still refractory. Statistically one might expect that a 50% chance existed for any anomalous beat to manifest a similar initial deflection as the normally conducted beats. A beat can only be directed in one of two ways (up or down). Consequently, detection of a similar initial deflection supports the diagnosis of aberrancy, but in no way rules out that the anomalous beat is a PVC. On the other hand, finding that the initial deflection of an anomalous beat is oppositely directed to the initial QRS vector of the normally conducted beats favors ventricular ectopy.

Diagnosis of aberrancy can be clinched by identification of a *premature* P wave in the T wave before the anomalous QRS complex. This premature P wave often is not as obvious as it is in Fig. 5-3 and may require close scrutiny and careful comparison with the normal T wave to detect it.

• • •

PROBLEM: Examine the rhythm strip shown in Fig. 5-4. This patient has a *wandering atrial pacemaker* as evidenced by a constantly changing PR interval and a variable P-wave morphology. The configuration of beat 9 significantly differs from that of the other QRS complexes and could easily be taken for a PVC. However, attention to the T wave preceding this beat reveals the telltale notching of a premature P wave. *Beat 9 is an aberrantly conducted PAC.* Are there any other premature P waves in this tracing?

ANSWER TO FIG. 5-4: Assuming that the T waves following beats 2, 3, 6, 7, and 11 in Fig. 5-4 are normal, all of the remaining T waves manifest some alteration in their morphology. (The T waves following beats 1, 5, and 10 are peaked, whereas the one after beat 4 is notched.) It would be easy to overlook these premature P waves if one failed to analyze T-wave morphology.

With the exception of beat 9, QRS complexes do not follow these premature P waves. PACs that occur early in the repolarization process during the absolute refractory period (ARP) (arrow A in Fig. 5-5) find the ventricles absolutely refractory to additional stimuli and will not be conducted (they are "blocked"). A PAC occurring somewhat later may arrive at the ventricles during the relative refractory period (RRP) (arrow B in Fig. 5-5) and find that a portion of the conduction system has recovered. Such a PAC may then conduct but

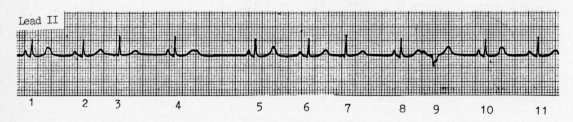

Fig. 5-4

with aberrancy, since the process of repolarization has not yet been completed. (This is the case with beat 9 in Fig. 5-4.) PACs occurring after complete recovery (arrow C in Fig. 5-5) are conducted normally to the ventricles.

• • •

PROBLEM: Check yourself on these concepts by looking at the rhythm strip shown in Fig. 5-6, taken from the MCL_1 lead of a patient in a bigeminal rhythm. There are two abnormal-looking complexes present, beats 2 and 6. Are these PVCs, or are they aberrantly conducted?

ANSWER TO FIG. 5-6: In Fig. 5-6 beats 2 and 6 manifest the three characteristic features of aberrancy that were already discussed: an initial deflection similar to that of the normally conducted beats, an RBBB pattern in a right-sided monitoring lead, and a premature P wave (which in this case is a tiny negative deflection with a short PR interval seen just before the onset of the QRS complex). These are *PJCs that conduct aberrantly*.

• • •

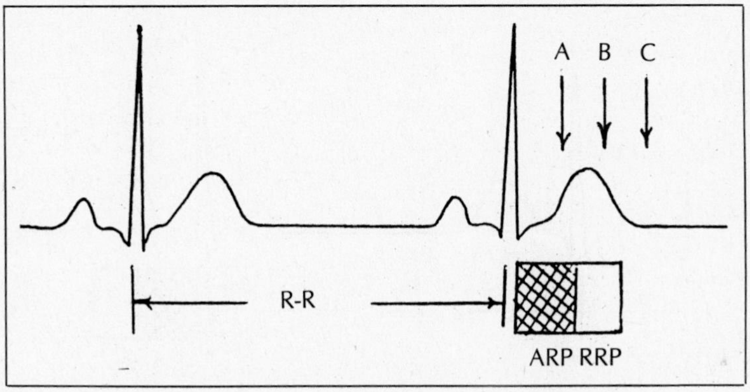

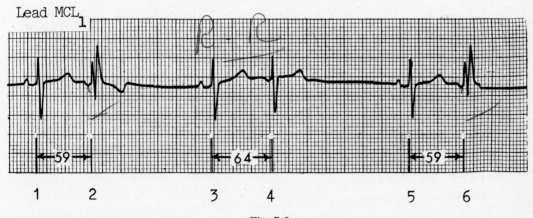

Fig. 5-5. Absolute and relative refractory periods.

Fig. 5-6

PROBLEM: Why does beat 4 not also conduct aberrantly?

ANSWER: Beat 4 conducts normally because it has a longer coupling interval than the aberrantly conducted beats. The *coupling interval* can be defined as the period between the R wave of one beat and the R wave of the subsequent premature beat. In Fig. 5-6 the coupling interval of beats 1 and 2 and 5 and 6 is .59 second, whereas the coupling interval for beats 3 and 4 is 0.64 second.

Beat 4 occurs at a time when the ventricles have recovered and corresponds to the impulse represented by arrow C in Fig. 5-5. In contrast, beats 2 and 6 occur during the RRP. They correspond to the impulse represented by arrow B in Fig. 5-5 and are conducted to the ventricles with aberrancy. Thus there is a *reason* for the aberrancy seen in Fig. 5-6; the premature beats that conduct aberrantly (beats 2 and 6) have a shorter coupling interval than the premature beat that conducts normally (beat 4).

ASHMAN PHENOMENON

In addition to the coupling interval, another important determinant of aberrancy is the R-R

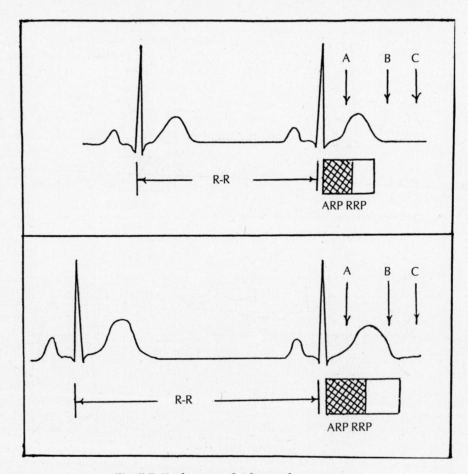

Fig. 5-7. Explanation of Ashman phenomenon.

interval that precedes the anomalous beat in question. This concept is explained by Fig. 5-7.

As previously discussed, premature impulses occuring during the ARP are blocked, whereas those that occur after repolarization is complete are conducted normally. Premature impulses occurring during the RRP conduct with aberrancy. Thus in the upper panel of Fig. 5-7 premature impulse A is blocked, but B and C are conducted normally.

The fact that the *duration of the total refractory period is directly proportional to the length of its preceding R-R interval* should now be considered. Thus when heart rate slows down, the R-R interval lengthens and the refractory period increases. This situation is illustrated in the lower panel of Fig. 5-7. With the increase in the R-R interval comes a corresponding increase in both the ARP and the RRP. Premature impulse A is still blocked, and impulse C is still conducted normally. However, impulse B, which previously occurred after the completion of repolarization, now occurs during the RRP and consequently is conducted with aberrancy. This is known as the *Ashman phenomenon,* which simply stated says that *the most aberrant beat is most likely to follow the longest pause.*

PROBLEM: Use the Ashman phenomenon to explain why beat 4 in Fig. 5-8 conducts aberrantly, whereas beat 6 does not.

ANSWER TO FIG. 5-8: Both of these beats (Fig. 5-8) occur prematurely with approximately the same coupling interval, yet the R-R interval preceding beat 4 (the R-R interval between beats 2 and 3) is clearly longer than the R-R interval preceding beat 6 (the R-R interval between beats 4 and 5). In other words, *the most aberrant beat* (beat 4) *follows the longest pause.*

COMPENSATORY PAUSES

The point has been made that finding a premature P wave in front of an abnormal-looking beat strongly suggests aberrancy. It should be emphasized that this P wave *must* be premature.

PROBLEM: For example, consider the rhythm strip shown in Fig. 5-9. Beat 4 is noticeably different from the other QRS complexes, yet it is preceded by a P wave. Is beat 4 a PVC, or is it an aberrantly conducted beat?

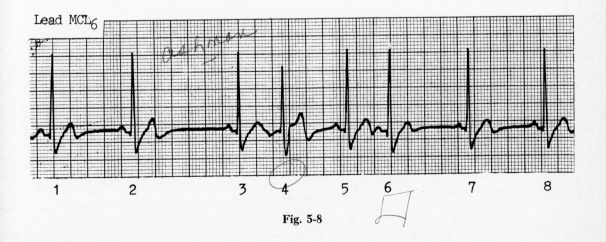

Fig. 5-8

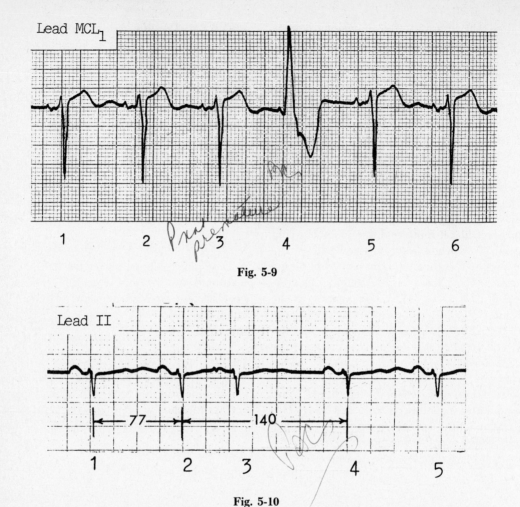

Lead MCL$_1$

Fig. 5-9

Lead II

Fig. 5-10

ANSWER TO FIG. 5-9: Beat 4 in Fig. 5-9 is a PVC. Although preceded by a P wave, this P wave is *not* premature. (If you set your calipers at the P-P interval between beats 2 and 3, you will find that the P wave preceding beat 4 is precisely on time.) Furthermore, the PR interval preceding beat 4 is far too short to conduct, implying that something must have occurred before the normal sinus-initiated impulse could stimulate the ventricles.

If you continue to walk out your calipers, you will find that the next P wave (the P wave preceding beat 5 in Fig. 5-9) also occurs precisely on time. PVCs usually do not conduct retrograde to the atria. Thus the SA node continues to fire uninterrupted, and P waves can be seen to "march on through." This accounts for why the pause containing the PVC in Fig. 5-9 (the interval from the R wave of beat 3 until the R wave of beat 5) is equal to twice the normal R-R interval (i.e., a *full compensatory pause* is present).

Conversely, PACs depolarize the atria and reset the sinus cycle. The pause containing a PAC therefore is usually not fully compensatory. The interval between beats 2 and 4 in Fig. 5-10 that contains the PAC (beat 3) is thus not equal to twice the regular sinus cycle.

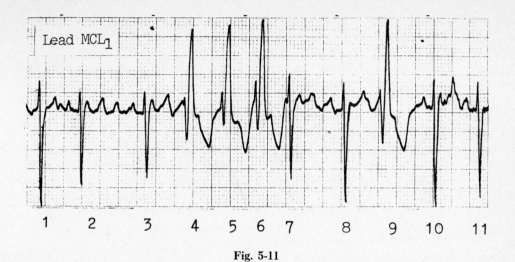

Fig. 5-11

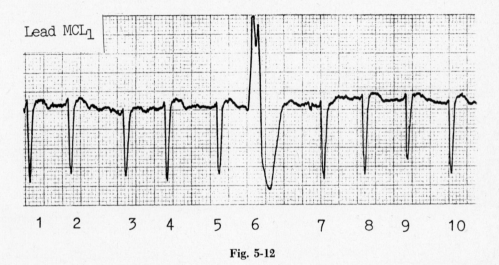

Fig. 5-12

Determining whether or not a full compensatory pause exists may be an additional helpful point in differentiating PVCs from aberrantly conducted beats. However, caution must be advised. PVCs *may* conduct retrograde to the atria, in which case they will reset the sinus cycle. Furthermore, a PAC can arise from a site in one of the atria that *by chance* lies at a distance such that the time required to depolarize the atria and reset the SA node coincidentally equals twice the normal R-R interval. Consequently, *PVCs do not always*

demonstrate a full compensatory pause, whereas PACs may occasionally do so. One cannot depend solely on the presence or absence of a compensatory pause but should rather use this information in the context of the other characteristics of the abnormal beat before deciding on its etiology.

QRS MORPHOLOGY

The final factor to consider in the differentiation of PVCs from aberrancy is the morphology of the QRS complex itself. As discussed, the finding of a *typical* RBBB pattern in a right-sided monitoring lead strongly suggests aberrancy. For example, the rhythm shown in Fig. 5-11 is taken from the MCL_1 lead of a patient in atrial flutter. Beats 4, 5, 6, and 9 are much more likely to be aberrantly conducted than ventricular ectopics. Each of these beats manifests an rSR′ configuration with a taller right "rabbit ear" (the R′ of each complex is taller than the initial r).

In contrast, beat 6 in Fig. 5-12 is a PVC in which the left rabbit ear is taller than the right. These and other morphologic features helpful in the differentiation of PVCs from aberrancy are summarized in Table 5-1.

Because the patient in Fig. 5-12 is in atrial fibrillation, a search for premature atrial activity does not help in determining whether beat 6 is a PVC or an aberrantly conducted beat. However, two other features support the diagnosis of ventricular ectopy. First, the QRS complex of beat 6 begins with a tiny negative deflection that is opposite to the initial positive deflection of the normally conducted beats. Second, the QRS duration of beat 6 is at least 0.16 second. *When QRS duration exceeds 0.14 second, ventricular ectopy is favored,* whereas a QRS duration of ≤ 0.12 second favors aberrancy.

A word of caution is in order. The appearance

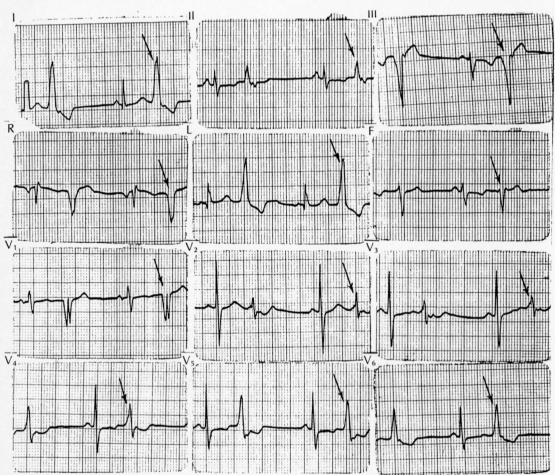

Fig. 5-13

Table 5-1. Features helpful in differentiating PVCs from aberrancy

ECG leads	Favors aberrancy	Favors ventricular ectopy	No help in differentiation
Morphologic features*			
V_1 or MCL_1	+++ rSR′ pattern with taller right rabbit ear	+++ R wave, qR, or slurred R wave with taller left rabbit ear	Slurred R wave with taller right rabbit ear
V_6 or MCL_6	++ qRS pattern (the reciprocal of the rSR′ in V_1)	++ QS or rS pattern	RS pattern
Other features*			
All leads	+ QRS duration ≤ 0.12	+ QRS duration > 0.14	
Any leads	+ Similar initial deflection of anomalous beats to normally conducted beats	++ Opposite initial deflection of anomalous beats to normally conducted beats	
Any leads	+++ Presence of *premature* P wave	+ Absence of premature P wave	
Any leads	+ Absence of compensatory pause	+ Presence of compensatory pause	
Any leads		+++ AV dissociation or fusion beats (Both are uncommon)	
All of the precordial leads (V_{1-6})		+++ Concordance of QRS vectors in *all* precordial leads (entirely upright or negative QRS complexes in leads V_{1-6}) (Uncommon)	

*+++Strongly, ++Moderately, +Slightly favoring.

of a PVC may vary markedly depending on which lead is used to monitor the patient. A premature beat that appears narrow (supraventricular) in one lead may look much wider and more bizarre (suggesting ventricular ectopy) when viewed from another lead.

Fig. 5-13 is taken from a patient who is in ventricular bigeminy. The arrows indicate the PVCs in each lead. The ectopic morphology varies in each of the 12 leads of the standard ECG. One certainly would have no difficulty identifying the PVCs in leads I, III, aVR, aVL, V_1, and V_6. The QRS is bizarre in shape and significantly wider than the normally conducted beats in each of these leads. The PVCs all demonstrate an oppositely directed initial QRS deflection, although this is not as obvious in leads I and aVL. (The normally conducted beats have a small septal q wave, whereas the PVCs begin with an oppositely directed upstroke in leads I and aVL.)

Identification of the bigeminal beats as PVCs is not nearly as apparent from inspection of leads II, aVF, V_2, and V_3. The initial deflection is identical to that of the normally conducted beats in these leads, and the QRS complex does not appear wide. Specifically, in leads V_2 and V_3 the normally conducted QRS complexes are of much greater amplitude than the beats that follow them and might be mistaken for PVCs if one did not see a P wave preceding them. Furthermore, notching in the T wave simulates a premature P wave in front of the PVCs in leads V_{3-6}.

DIFFERENTIATION OF PVCS FROM ABERRANCY WITH ATRIAL FIBRILLATION

Differentiation of PVCs from aberrancy is especially difficult in the setting of atrial fibrillation. The reason is twofold. First, because of the loss of organized atrial activity, P waves are no longer evident on the ECG. Consequently, the important differentiating feature of identifying a premature P wave is lost.

Second, the Ashman phenomenon is of uncertain validity in the presence of atrial fibrillation,

since the length of the R-R interval is constantly being influenced by concealed conduction and no longer accurately reflects the duration of the subsequent refractory period.

PROBLEM: We can partially compensate for these drawbacks by profiting from the irregularity that is inherent in atrial fibrillation. For example, examine the abnormal-appearing beats in Figs. 5-14 and 5-15 taken from two patients who are completely asymptomatic. Is ventricular ectopy likely to be present in one or both of these tracings?

ANSWER TO FIG. 5-14: In Fig. 5-14 there is a string of seven abnormally wide beats that at least initially suggests a run of ventricular tachycardia. However, the rhythm remains irregularly irregular throughout the entire strip irrespective of the width of the QRS complex. Since *ventricular tachycardia is usually a fairly regular rhythm*, the gross irregularity present here favors aberrancy, although one cannot be certain from this tracing alone. Analysis of QRS morphology is not helpful in differentiation of PVCs from aberrancy in a standard lead II as was used here. The patient remained asymptomatic and demonstrated wide complexes with a typical aberrant morphology when switched to a right sided lead.

ANSWER TO FIG. 5-15: Atrial fibrillation is again evident from the lack of P waves and the erratic baseline (Fig. 5-15). A wide and bizarre QRS complex occurs every other beat, but whereas the underlying rhythm is irregularly irregular, the coupling interval of each bigeminal beat is fixed. This suggests that these beats are PVCs, since one would expect aberrantly conducted beats to also be irregular when the underlying rhythm is atrial fibrillation. Other factors favoring ventricular ectopy are the width of this QRS complex (which is at least 0.15 second) and a "q-slur-R" configuration of the QRS with a taller left rabbit ear and

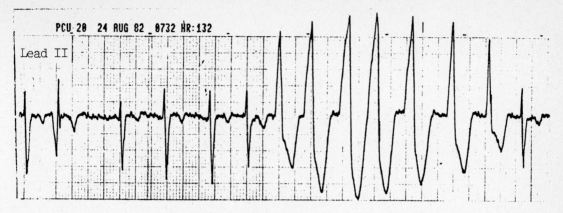

PCU 20 24 AUG 82 0732 HR:132

Lead II

Fig. 5-14

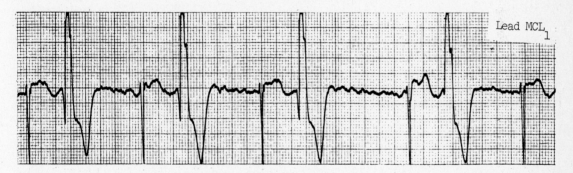

Lead MCL$_1$

Fig. 5-15

an initial negative deflection that is opposite that of the normally conducted beats. The patient was treated with lidocaine.

• • •

PROBLEM: As review, return to the question posed at the beginning of this chapter as to whether ventricular ectopy is present in Fig. 5-1 and/or Fig. 5-2.

ANSWER: It should be clear that the two abnormal beats in Fig. 5-2 are PVCs. Although the initial deflection of these beats is similar to that of the normally conducted complexes, the duration of the QRS complex is greatly

prolonged (to ≥ 0.15 second), and P waves can be seen to walk right through the tracing, resulting in a perfectly compensatory pause. The P wave seen before the second of these abnormal beats cannot be a PAC that conducts aberrantly, since the PR interval is too short to conduct, and the P wave is not premature. The QRS configuration is of an rS pattern that also suggests ventricular ectopy in this left sided lead.

On the other hand, the three abnormal beats that appear in succession in Fig. 5-1 are aberrantly conducted. The three most helpful features for identifying aberrancy are evident: an RBBB pattern, an initial deflection similar to that of the normally conducted beats, and a premature P wave that can be seen to produce a notch in the T wave immediately preceding the triplet. The underlying rhythm is multifocal atrial tachycardia (MAT) with an irregularly irregular rhythm but manifesting well-defined (albeit different) P waves in front of most QRS complexes. Finally, the Ashman phenomenon is present (the first aberrant beat in the tracing follows the longest pause).

SUGGESTED READINGS

Langendorf, R, Pick, A, and Winternitz, M: Mechanisms of intermittent ventricular bigeminy. I. Appearance of ectopic beats dependent upon length of the ventricular cycle, the "Rule of Bigeminy," Circulation 11:422-430, 1955.

Marriott, H.J.L.: Practical electrocardiography, Baltimore, 1982, The Williams & Wilkins Co.

Marriott, H.J.L., and Conover, M.H.B.: Advanced concepts in arrhythmias, St. Louis, 1983, The C.V. Mosby Co.

Swanick, E.J., LaCamera, F., and Marriott, H.J.L.: Morphologic features of right ventricular ectopic beats, Am. J. Cardiol. 30:888-891, 1972.

Vera, Z., Cheng, T.O., Ertem, G., Shoaleh-var, M., Wickramasekaran, R., and Wadhwa, K.: His bundle electrography for evaluation of criteria in differentiating ventricular ectopy from aberrancy in atrial fibrillation (abstract), Circulation 45-46 (supp. 2):90, 1972.

Wellens, H.J.J., Bar, F.W.H.M., and Lie, K.I.: The value of the electrocardiogram in the differential diagnosis of a tachycardia with a widened QRS complex, Am. J. Med. 64:27-33, 1978.

CHAPTER 6

Tachydysrhythmias

Perhaps the greatest challenge faced by the emergency care provider during cardiac resuscitation is the task of interpreting tachydysrhythmias. Institution of the appropriate treatment and the ultimate fate of the patient often hang in the balance.

The goal of this chapter is to incorporate the material covered in the previous two chapters on rate, rhythm, and aberrancy into a working plan for approaching the tachydysrhythmias as they may occur in an emergency care setting.

PROBLEM: Consider first the problem posed by a middle-aged patient with the tachydysrhythmia shown in Fig. 6-1. How would you proceed both diagnostically and therapeutically if the patient were tolerating this rhythm?

ANSWER TO FIG. 6-1: A regular tachydysrhythmia with a rate of about 200 beats/min is seen in Fig. 6-1. No distinct P waves can be identified. The critical question is whether this represents SVT or ventricular tachycardia. The answer is not forthcoming from analysis of this single rhythm strip. One cannot tell if the QRS complex is widened, since it is virtually impossible to be sure where the QRS complex ends and the ST segment begins. Even if the QRS complex were wide, the possibility would exist that this is SVT with preexisting bundle branch block or aberrant conduction.

Practically speaking, one is left with three alternatives.

1. *Seek more information.*
   a. Obtain a 12-lead ECG to see if P waves are evident in any other leads or if QRS morphology can aid in differentiation. (See Table 5-1.)
   b. Determine if rhythm strips are available on the patient before he went into the tachycardia. Is the QRS configuration during sinus rhythm similar to that shown in Fig. 6-1? (If so, this implies a supraventricular etiology for the rhythm. If not, the question still remains as to whether Fig. 6-1 represents ventricular tachycardia or a supraventricular dysrhythmia with aberrancy).
   c. Look at the neck veins and listen to the first heart sound. The presence of irregular cannon waves in the neck and/or variation in the intensity of the first heart sound suggests AV dissociation and supports the diagnosis of ventricular tachycardia (but does not rule out the possibility of AV dissociation between an atrial and junctional pacemaker). A lack of variation in the intensity of the first heart sound and either the absence of cannon waves or the presence of regular cannon waves in the neck are evi-

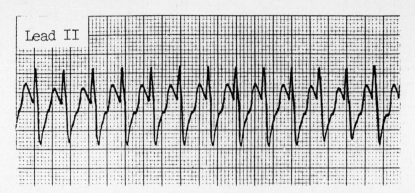

Fig. 6-1. From Grauer, K., and Curry, R.W., Jr.: Monograph 47, AAFP Home Study Self-Assessment, © 1983, American Academy of Family Physicians.

dence against AV dissociation. This suggests a supraventricular etiology of the tachydysrhythmia (but does not rule out ventricular tachycardia with 1:1 retrograde conduction).

2. *Assume the rhythm to be supraventricular, and treat accordingly.* This would be reasonable, since the QRS complex looks like it is probably not very much widened and the patient is tolerating the dysrhythmia, which in conjunction with a heart rate of about 200 beats/min favors a supraventricular etiology. (However, *patients with ventricular tachycardia may occasionally remain conscious and alert for extended periods of time.*)

a. Apply *CSM*. Under constant ECG monitoring, turn the patient's head to the left, and gently but firmly massage the area of the right carotid bifurcation near the angle of the jaw for 5 seconds at a time. After several attempts on the right carotid, the other side may be tried. (*Never* massage both sides simultaneously.)

The response to CSM varies depending on the nature of the dysrhythmia. The most dramatic response occurs with PSVT in which

CSM may abruptly terminate the tachycardia. Alternatively, PSVT may not respond at all to the maneuver. Ventricular tachycardia does not respond to CSM. Consequently, a lack of response to CSM would not differentiate between these two dysrhythmias. (See Table 6-1 for the expected response of these and other dysrhythmias to CSM).

CSM is not a totally benign maneuver, particularly in older individuals; it has been associated with syncope, stroke, sinus arrest, high-grade AV block, prolonged asystole, and ventricular tachydysrhythmias in patients with digitalis intoxication. As a result, it should probably not be attempted in patients with a history of SSS, cervical bruits, or cerebrovascular disease, or when the possibility of digitalis intoxication exists.

b. Administer IV verapamil. This drug has become the favored treatment for PSVT, successfully converting it to sinus rhythm over 90% of the time. A dose of 5 to 10 mg (i.e., 0.075-0.150 mg/kg) is given IV over a 1- to 2-minute period and repeated if needed in 30 minutes. (However,

Table 6-1. Effects of carotid sinus massage on tachydysrhythmias

Tachydysrhythmias	Response to CSM
Sinus tachycardia	Gradual slowing with CSM with resumption of the tachycardia after the maneuver
PSVT—PAT, PJT	Abrupt termination of the tachydysrhythmia with conversion to sinus rhythm, *or* No response to CSM
Atrial flutter or atrial fibrillation	Increased degree of AV block with resultant slowing of the ventricular rate (CSM often permits diagnosis of atrial flutter by allowing clear visualization of flutter waves as the ventricular rate slows)
Ventricular tachycardia	No response to CSM

verapamil should not be used indiscriminately as a diagnostic maneuver to differentiate SVT from ventricular tachycardia in cases of wide-complex tachydysrhythmias, since the drug may cause deterioration of ventricular tachycardia to ventricular fibrillation.)

Second-line drugs for treatment of PSVT include digoxin and propranolol. Digoxin would *not* be recommended in this case, since the possibility still exists that the rhythm in Fig. 6-1 is ventricular tachycardia for which digitalis is contraindicated. Propanolol may be effective for both supraventricular or ventricular tachydysrhythmias, but the IV form of this drug should not be given soon after verapamil, since this increases the risk of inducing AV block.

  c. If the patient at any time shows signs of hemodynamic decompensation, cardioversion should immediately be employed.

3. *Assume the rhythm to be ventricular tachycardia and treat accordingly.*
  a. Give the patient a bolus of lidocaine, and begin an IV infusion.
  b. Begin cardioversion; this modality should be effective regardless of whether the rhythm in Fig. 6-1 is supraventricular or ventricular in nature. As long as the patient is tolerating the dysrhythmia, cardioversion may be done under semielective conditions. The patient may be sedated with 5 to 10 mg of IV valium, anesthesiologists can be called to the bedside, and lower energy levels (20 to 50 J) may be tried first.

This example emphasizes the difficulty that may exist in differentiating supraventricular from ventricular tachydysrhythmias when the QRS complex appears wide. The ramifications of this diagnostic dilemma on treatment are obvious.

NARROW COMPLEX TACHYDYSRHYTHMIAS

Classification of tachydysrhythmias is much easier when the QRS complex is of normal duration. In this case evaluation of the rhythm's regularity and identification of atrial activity become the important differentiating factors.

PROBLEM: Use this information to interpret the supraventricular tachydysrhythmias shown in Figs. 6-2 to 6-6, all taken from lead II monitoring leads.

ANSWER TO FIG. 6-2: In Fig. 6-2 the rhythm is regular at a rate of about 125 beats/min. Normal upright P waves with a PR interval of

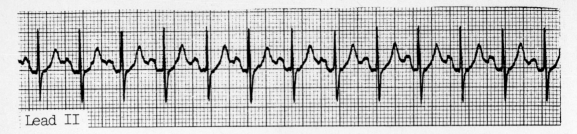

Lead II

Fig. 6-2

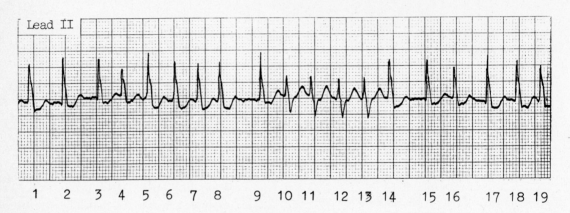

Lead II

1   2   3   4   5   6   7   8   9   10 11   12 13 14   15 16   17 18 19

Fig. 6-3

about 0.16 second precede each QRS complex. This is *sinus tachycardia*.

ANSWER TO FIG. 6-3: The rhythm is irregularly irregular, and no P waves are evident in Fig. 6-3. This is *atrial fibrillation* with a *rapid ventricular response* (the mean ventricular rate is faster than 120 beats/min.)

• • •

PROBLEM: Are beats 10 to 13 in Fig. 6-3 PVCs or aberrantly conducted beats?

ANSWER: Beats 10 to 13 in Fig. 6-3 are aberrantly conducted. The QRS duration of these beats is only minimally prolonged (to about 0.11 second), they have an initial deflection similar to that of the normally conducted

beats, and they maintain the same irregularity of the underlying rhythm. The Ashman phenomenon is present (the first beat in the run of aberrant beats begins following the longest pause), although as previously mentioned, this criterion is of less diagnostic significance in the presence of atrial fibrillation.

ANSWER TO FIG. 6-4: Once again the rhythm is irregularly irregular (Fig. 6-4). As opposed to Fig. 6-3 in which no atrial activity is evident, definite P waves precede many of the QRS complexes in Fig. 6-4. Some of these P waves are positive (the P waves preceding beats 2 to 4, and 6 to 12); others are biphasic (the P waves preceding beats 13 and 14) or negative (the P waves preceding beats 1 and 15 to 17). The PR interval constantly varies. No P wave

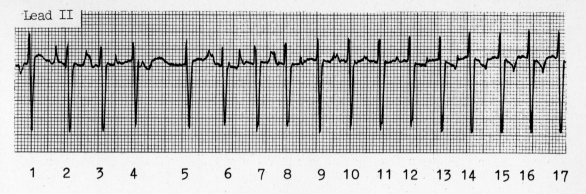

Fig. 6-4

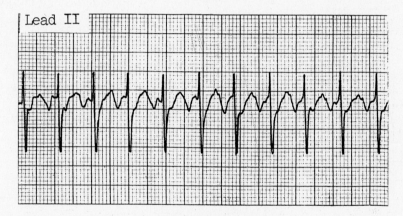

Fig. 6-5

precedes beat 5, and a blocked PAC notches the T wave of beat 4. This is *MAT (multifocal atrial tachycardia)*.

MAT is most often seen among patients with chronic obstructive pulmonary disease. It is important clinically to distinguish this dysrhythmia from atrial fibrillation, since treatment of these two entities dramatically differs. With rapid atrial fibrillation, digitalization constitutes the medical treatment of choice. The ventricular response can be used to gauge the amount of intravenous digoxin that needs to be administered. Following an initial loading dose of between 0.50 and 0.75 mg of digoxin, increments of 0.125 to 0.250

mg can be given every few hours until the ventricular response is under control.

Conversely, treatment of MAT must be directed to correcting the underlying cause of the dysrhythmia (hypoxemia). MAT is notoriously resistant to treatment with digoxin. It is easy to imagine what might happen if one fails to recognize this dysrhythmia and embarks on a course of digitalization. Not surprisingly, digitalis toxicity is one of the leading causes of mortality in patients with MAT.

ANSWER TO FIG. 6-5: The rhythm in Fig. 6-5 is regular at a rate of just over 150 beats/min. A *negative* deflection precedes each QRS com-

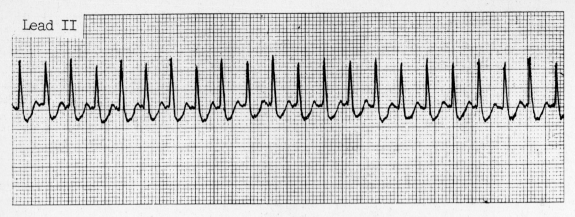

Fig. 6-6

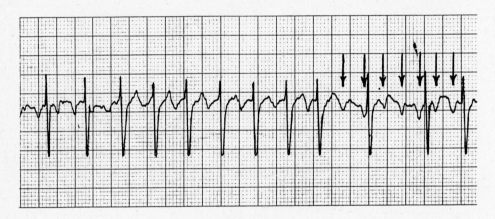

Fig. 6-7

plex. This cannot represent normal atrial activity, since *sinus-initiated P waves must always be upright in lead II*. Possibilities to include in the differential diagnosis are PAT or PJT but *with a ventricular response in the vicinity of 150 beats/min, a diagnosis of atrial flutter should be strongly considered*.

ANSWER TO FIG. 6-6: Fig. 6-6 illustrates a regular SVT at a rate of 220 beats/min. It is too fast to be sinus tachycardia. Atrial flutter is also unlikely, since the atrial rate would have to be 440 beats/min if 2:1 AV conduction were present. The rhythm could be atrial flutter with 1:1 AV conduction, but this would require an atrial rate of 220 beats/min, some-

thing that is unlikely unless the patient were taking a medication such as quinidine that slows the atrial response. The most probable diagnosis therefore is either *PAT* or *PJT*. Differentiation between these two possibilities is impossible, since P waves cannot be identified at this rate.

• • •

PROBLEM: Returning to the rhythm shown in Fig. 6-5, what maneuver might help to confirm the diagnosis of atrial flutter?

ANSWER: *CSM* might help to confirm the diagnosis of atrial flutter. Fig. 6-7 demonstrates

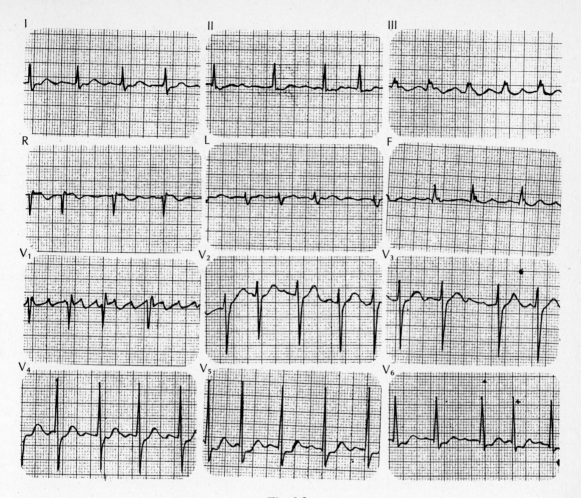

Fig. 6-8

how increasing the degree of AV block by CSM uncovers telltale flutter waves (arrows) that could not be detected when the rate was faster.

Flutter waves may at times be seen in some monitoring leads but not in others. Even with the benefit of a 12-lead ECG, the diagnosis can be subtle. For example, consider the ECG shown in Fig. 6-8.

An irregularly irregular rhythm is apparent that at first glance seems to be atrial fibrillation with a controlled ventricular response. No atrial activity is observed anywhere on the tracing until attention is directed to precordial lead V_1 where the characteristic sawtooth configuration of *atrial flutter* is evident. Whereas the ventricular response is most often regular in atrial flutter at a rate of about 150 beats/min, a variable ventricular response may occur (as shown here), and more than one monitoring lead may be needed to detect occult flutter waves. Atrial flutter is perhaps the one rhythm that most often requires a high index of suspicion to make the diagnosis.

Lead II

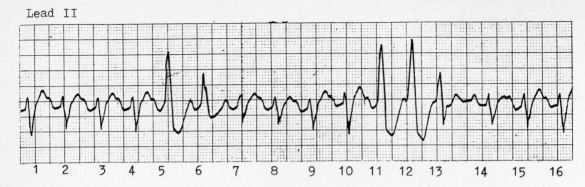

Fig. 6-9

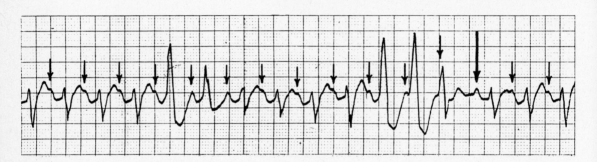

Fig. 6-10

IDENTIFICATION OF ATRIAL ACTIVITY

Detection of P waves in a tachydysrhythmia and determination of the relationship of these P waves to the QRS complex are of enormous benefit in rhythm interpretation.

PROBLEM: Try interpreting the next two examples, beginning with Fig. 6-9.

ANSWER TO FIG. 6-9: The basic rhythm in Fig. 6-9 is composed of rS complexes that are slightly widened (beats 1 to 4, 7 to 10, and 14 to 16). It is fairly regular at a rate of about 125 beats/min. A number of wider, predominantly positive QRS deflections are also seen in the tracing (beats 5, 6, and 11 to 13). Atrial activity is not evident *except* before beat 14. As a result of a slowing of the underlying rhythm, a well-defined P wave with a PR

interval of 0.21 second can be seen to precede this beat. Setting one's calipers to the R-R interval and beginning at the peak of this P wave, atrial activity can be "marched out" across the entire rhythm strip (Fig. 6-11). It now becomes evident that the underlying rhythm is *sinus tachycardia*. Because of the rapid rate, P waves are hidden within the ST segment and notch the terminal portion of the T wave. Beats 5, 6, and 11 to 13 must therefore be PCVs, since they are wide and are not related to the atrial activity (there is AV dissociation).

ANSWER TO FIG. 6-10: In Fig. 6-10 the basic rhythm is composed of QS complexes that are 0.12 second in duration and regular at a rate of 135 beats/min. Two "unusual" complexes

Lead II

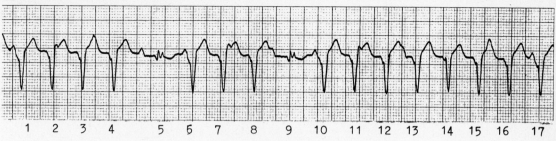

Fig. 6-11

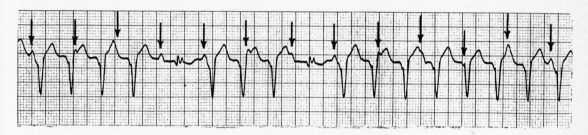

Fig. 6-12

(beats 5 and 9) interrupt this underlying rhythm. Beat 5 is preceded by a P wave that appears to be conducting, although with first-degree AV block. Scanning the rest of the tracing for signs of atrial activity, notching and peaking at various points of the QRS complex in many beats are evident. Setting one's calipers to the interval defined by the P wave preceding beat 5 and the positive deflection that occurs just before beat 6, atrial activity can again be "marched out" throughout the rhythm strip (Fig. 6-12). This atrial activity is unrelated to the negative QRS complexes. Thus *AV dissociation* exists, with the negative QRS complexes representing runs of ventricular tachycardia that are interrupted by *sinus capture beats* (beats 5 and 9). The q waves of these sinus beats and the first-degree AV

block are manifestations of the patient's acute inferior myocardial infarction.

The finding of *AV dissociation* during a wide-complex tachycardia is extremely useful in identifying the tachydysrhythmia as being ventricular in origin. Although it is theoretically possible that AV dissociation may be the result of an aberrantly conducted accelerated junctional pacemaker, ventricular tachycardia is statistically much more likely. Unfortunately, this helpful diagnostic feature is only seen in a minority of cases of ventricular tachycardia.

• • •

Lead V_1

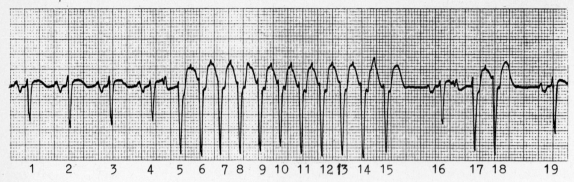

Fig. 6-13

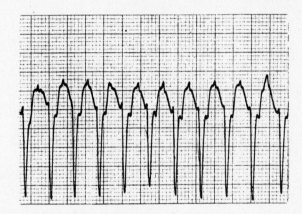

Fig. 6-14

PROBLEM: Finally, examine the rhythm in Fig. 6-13. Sinus tachycardia at a rate of 100 beats/min is seen for the first four beats. This is interrupted by a tachydysrhythmia (beats 5 to 15) with a wider and deeper QRS configuration and a rate of 220 beats/min. Is this a run of ventricular tachycardia, or is it SVT with aberrant conduction?

ANSWER TO FIG. 6-13: Fig. 6-13 illustrates the importance of catching a tachydysrhythmia at its onset. Imagine that all one had captured was the tachydysrhythmia itself (Fig. 6-14).

Although the QRS complex is only minimally widened and the rapid rate would favor a supraventricular etiology, one could not absolutely rule out ventricular tachycardia on the basis of the rhythm strip shown in Fig. 6-14 alone. The tiny positive deflections seen at the peak of each T wave suggest atrial activity but are of no assistance in differentiation, since they could represent either antegrade atrial activation or retrograde atrial activation arising from the AV node (as in SVT) or from the ventricles (as in ventricular tachycardia).

However, if we return to Fig. 6-13 and direct our attention to the T wave just preceding the onset of the tachydysrhythmia, a notched premature P wave becomes apparent. Similarly, one beat after termination of the tachydysrhythmia, a premature P wave is seen to deform the T wave of beat 16, resulting in aberration of beats 17 and 18. These PACs (beats 17 and 18) are identical to the

Lead II

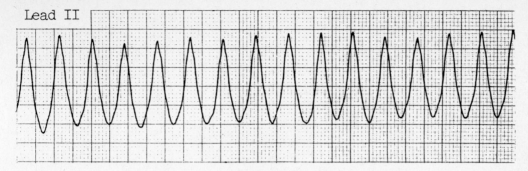

Fig. 6-15

Lead II

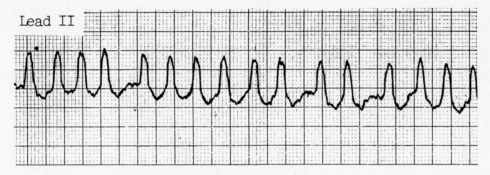

Fig. 6-16

QRS configuration during the tachydysrhythmia. This confirms that beats 5 to 15 are the result of *aberrant conduction*.

It was previously stressed that most aberrantly conducted beats manifest an RBBB pattern. Fig. 6-13 is interesting in that the rSR′ pattern that we are accustomed to seeing in right-sided leads with aberrant conduction is not present. Instead, the aberration in this figure is of the left bundle branch block (LBBB) type. In addition to being much less common than the RBBB type, LBBB aberration is often more difficult to differentiate from ventricular ectopy.

WIDE COMPLEX TACHYDYSRHYTHMIAS

This chapter is completed by examining some additional examples of wide complex tachydysrhythmias.

PROBLEM: How would you interpret the rhythms shown in Figs. 6-15 to 6-17?

ANSWER TO FIG. 6-15: A regular wide complex tachydysrhythmia is present in Fig. 6-15 at a rate of 170 beats/min. No atrial activity is evident. This is *ventricular tachycardia* until proven otherwise.

ANSWER TO FIG. 6-16: A wide complex tachydysrhythmia is present in Fig. 6-16 that superficially resembles ventricular tachycardia. However, the rhythm is irregularly irregular, and no P waves can be identified. This is *atrial fibrillation* with a *rapid ventricular response*. Prolongation of the QRS complex can be explained either on the basis of rate-related aberrancy or preexisting bundle branch block.

Lead V_6

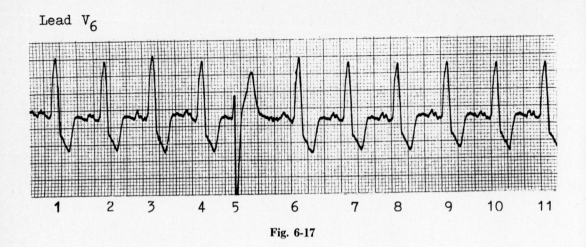

Fig. 6-17

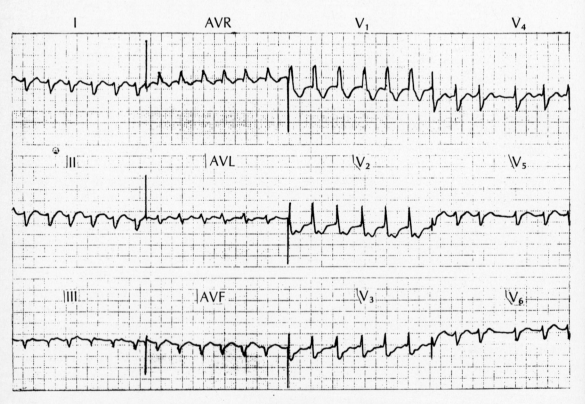

Fig. 6-18

ANSWER TO FIG. 6-17: Again the QRS complex is wide in Fig. 6-17, but the rhythm is regular at 100 beats/min and each complex (with the exception of beat 5) is preceded by a P wave. This is *sinus tachycardia* with *preexisting LBBB*. Beat 5 is a PVC.

• • •

PROBLEM: Twelve-lead ECGs of the last two patients are shown in Figs. 6-18 and 6-19. Each was known to have a history of some type of bundle branch block. Is either of them in ventricular tachycardia?

ANSWER TO FIG. 6-18: A wide complex tachydysrhythmia is present in Fig. 6-18 that superficially resembles ventricular tachycardia. No P waves can be identified. The rhythm appears to be fairly regular for most of the ECG; however, the gross irregularity evident in leads V_{4-6} is a tip-off that this is *atrial fibrillation*. QRS prolongation is the result of coexistence of RBBB and left anterior hemiblock.

ANSWER TO FIG. 6-19: A regular wide complex tachydysrhythmia at a rate of 125 beats/min is present in Fig. 6-19 that superficially resembles LBBB. However, the QRS morphology in the precordial leads is *not* typical for LBBB. As previously indicated in Table 5-1, finding concordance of the QRS vectors in the precordial leads (global positivity or negativity of the QRS complex in leads V_{1-6}) and a QS or rS configuration in lead V_6 (instead of the normal upright QRS configuration in this lead) strongly favors ventricular ectopy. This is *ventricular tachycardia*.

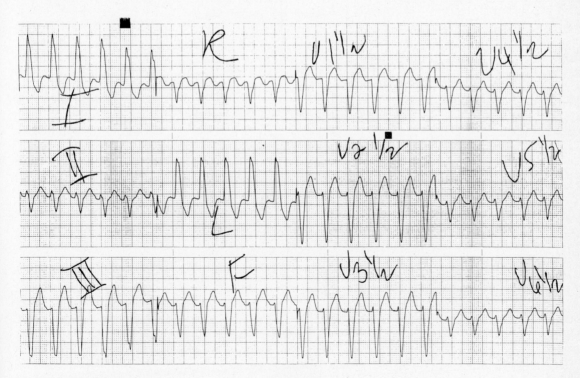

Fig. 6-19

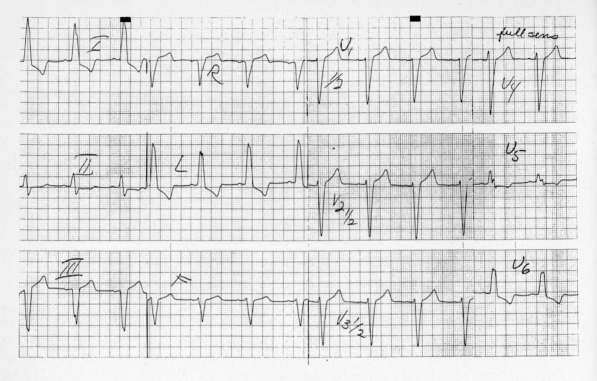

Fig. 6-20

Fig. 6-20 is taken from the same patient following cardioversion. Sinus rhythm has been restored as evidenced by normal-appearing P waves in front of all QRS complexes. LBBB is present. Whereas the QRS configuration of the limb leads is not significantly altered from what it was while the patient was in ventricular tachycardia, the QRS complex is now upright in lead V_6.

Although many of the rhythms used in this chapter are subtle examples of the various supraventricular and ventricular tachydysrhythmias, they emphasize the need for maintaining a high index of suspicion during interpretation and for paying careful attention to rate, regularity of rhythm, width of the QRS complex, and the presence or absence of atrial activity with its relationship to the QRS complex.

SUGGESTED READINGS

Chung, E.K.: Electrocardiography: practical applications with vectorial principles, New York, 1980, Harper & Row, Publishers, Inc., pp. 305-328.

Marriott, H.J.L.: Practical electrocardiography, Baltimore, 1982, The Williams & Wilkins Co.

Marriott, H.J.L., and Conover, M.H.B.: Advanced concepts in arrhythmias, St. Louis, 1983, The C.V. Mosby Co.

CHAPTER 7

AV block

There is probably no area in dysrhythmia interpretation that has generated as much controversy and confusion as the AV blocks. Disagreement commences with the terminology, encompasses diagnosis, and extends into therapeutic implications.

The goal of this chapter is to review the distinctions between the various types of AV blocks and to present a simplified method for arriving at their correct diagnosis. The decision-making process used is summarized in Algorithm G on p. 100. Referral to this figure while reading the chapter may be helpful in conceptualizing the material.

The boxed material on this page indicates the traditional classification of the AV blocks. Implicit in the division of these blocks into three degrees is the assumption that second-degree block portends a more ominous prognosis than first-degree block and that third-degree block portends the poorest prognosis of all. This is not necessarily the case.

In addition, terms such as *high-degree* or *high-grade heart block* and *AV dissociation* do not fit neatly into the classification. For instance, with third-degree AV block there is complete AV dissociation, but AV dissociation frequently occurs without third-degree AV block.

FIRST- AND THIRD-DEGREE AV BLOCK

First-degree AV block is easy to recognize. All atrial impulses are conducted to the ventricles

---

CLASSIFICATION OF AV BLOCK

First-degree AV block
Second-degree AV block
   Mobitz I (Wenckebach)
   Mobitz II
Third-degree AV block (i.e., complete heart block)

AV dissociation?
High-grade heart block?
High-degree block?

---

but with a prolonged PR interval (PR > 0.20 second). This is the case in Fig. 7-1 in which the atrial and ventricular rates are regular at 65 beats/min. Each QRS complex is preceded by a P wave with a constant PR interval that is prolonged to 0.34 second.

In *third-degree AV (complete) block* none of the atrial impulses are able to penetrate through to the ventricles. This results in a complete separation of atrial activity from the rest of the conduction system. For example, in Fig. 7-2 the SA node continues to fire at a rate of 100 beats/min, but P waves "march through" the QRS complex without any relation to the ventricular response. This phenomenon is known as *complete AV dissociation* and is easily recognized by the *varying PR interval*. With third-degree heart block, then, one would expect a constant atrial rate

91

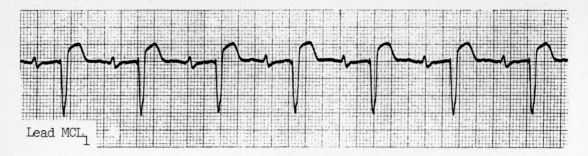

Lead MCL₁

Fig. 7-1

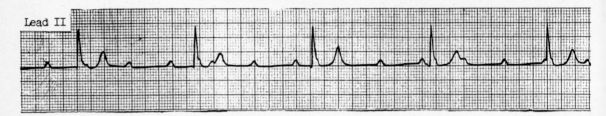

Lead II

Fig. 7-2

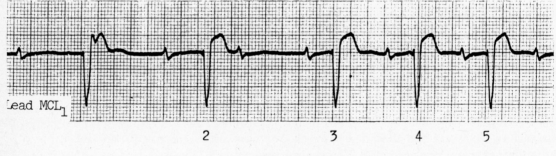

Lead MCL₁

2   3   4   5

Fig. 7-3

(regular P-P interval) and a constant ventricular rate (regular R-R interval) but no relation between the two.

Most of the time the ventricular response is regular with third-degree AV block. This is a helpful feature to look for when sorting out AV conduction disturbances, since recognition of R-R irregularity usually eliminates complete AV block from the differential.

PROBLEM: Fig. 7-3 is taken from the same patient who was shown to be in first-degree AV block in Fig. 7-1. Initially in this tracing, P waves appear to be totally unrelated to the QRS complex. Is third-degree AV block present?

ANSWER TO FIG. 7-3: Third-degree AV block is *not* present in Fig. 7-3, since AV conduction with first-degree AV block is able to resume

Lead II

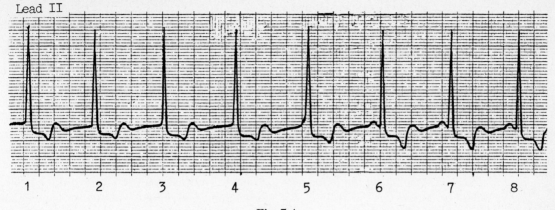

Fig. 7-4

Lead MCL₁

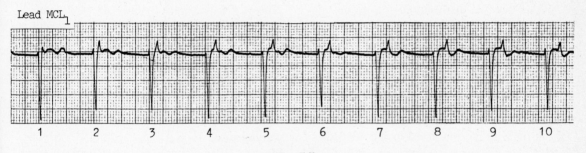

Fig. 7-5

later in the tracing. Instead there is *transient AV dissociation*. We can recognize at a glance that third-degree AV block is probably not present in Fig. 7-3 because the ventricular rate does not remain constant.

Consider the rhythm shown in Fig. 7-4. This tracing begins with a junctional rhythm at 70 beats/min. As the junctional pacemaker slows down ever so slightly, P waves can be seen to emerge from the QRS complex, beginning with the P wave that deforms the upstroke of the QRS complex of beat 5. This atrial pacemaker is set at 68 beats/min and ultimately takes over but initially is unrelated to the more rapid junctional pacemaker (i.e., the PR interval of beat 5 is definitely too short to conduct). Transient AV dissociation is again present but this time the mechanism is dif-

ferent. Because of acceleration of the AV nodal pacemaker to a rate of 70 beats/min during the first portion of this rhythm strip, *AV dissociation* occurs *by usurpation* of the rhythm from the sinus pacemaker. Alternatively, AV dissociation may also occur by *default* when the sinus pacemaker slows down and its function is taken over by a junctional or ventricular escape focus that is not accelerated.

Finally, examine the junctional rhythm illustrated in Fig. 7-5.

Complete AV dissociation is present in Fig. 7-5, since atrial activity is totally unrelated to the QRS complex. That is, the R-P interval varies, progressively lengthening from beat 1 to beat 10. The atrial rate itself is constant at 72 beats/min, but this is a bit slower than the junctional rate. When atrial and junctional pacemakers operate at nearly identical rates as shown here, the condition is known as *isorhythmic AV dissociation*.

The important point to make from Fig. 7-5 is that despite the presence of complete AV dissociation, it is impossible to determine whether or not third-degree AV block exists, since *the opportunity for normal sinus conduction never arises*. P waves always occur during the refractory period and should not be expected to conduct to the ventricles. Thus *before diagnosis of complete AV block is made, all of the following conditions should be looked for:*

- Regularity of the atrial rate
- Regularity of the ventricular rate
- Complete AV dissociation despite an adequate opportunity for normal conduction to occur

This last condition implies that the ventricular rate must be slow enough (and the rhythm strip long enough) for P waves to occur beyond the reaches of the refractory period and at points during the R-R interval at which one would expect them to be conducted to the ventricles. This usually requires a ventricular rate of 45 beats/min or less. Attention to this factor is critical in avoiding the overdiagnosis of conditions such as AV dissociation by usurpation (Fig. 7-5) as complete AV block.

The prognosis and need for treatment of AV dissociation depend on the severity of the underlying conduction disorder. In Fig. 7-5 usurpation of the normal sinus pacemaker by an accelerated junctional rhythm appears to be the mechanism responsible for the dysrhythmia. No specific treatment other than looking for the cause of the junctional tachycardia would be indicated, since the rate of the escape pacemaker is adequate. In contrast, treatment of the rhythm shown in Fig. 7-3 with atropine; infusion of dopamine, epinephrine, or isoproterenol; and/or pacemaker insertion would have to be strongly considered in this example of AV dissociation in which a more severe conduction disturbance is likely.

SECOND-DEGREE AV BLOCK

If the atrial rate is *regular* and some of the atrial impulses are conducted through to the ventricles but others are not, *second-degree AV block* exists. It is important to emphasize the need for *regularity of the atrial rate* in this definition. An awareness of this point helps to differentiate second-degree AV blocks from mimics such as blocked PACs and sinus pauses. In addition, consideration must be given to the appropriateness of the failed conduction. For example, the usual atrial rate in flutter is 300 beats/min. One-to-one ventricular conduction under these circumstances would be incompatible with life. Fortunately, the AV node is able to protect the ventricles by only allowing conduction of every other atrial impulse. The result is that the most common ventricular response in atrial flutter is approximately 150 beats/min. This rhythm should not be misclassified as a type of 2:1 AV block. Rather it represents physiologic 2:1 AV conduction.

The second-degree AV blocks have been divided into Mobitz I and Mobitz II varieties. *Mobitz I (Wenckebach) second-degree AV block* is characterized by progressive lengthening of the PR interval until a beat is dropped. In Fig. 7-6 the PR interval of beat 1 is 0.26 second. This lengthens to a PR interval of 0.44 second by beat 2, after which the next P wave is dropped. The cycle resumes with a PR interval of 0.24 second for the third QRS complex (beat 3). There are three P waves for each two QRS complexes throughout this rhythm strip (there is *3:2 AV conduction*).

Mobitz I second-degree AV block is most often associated with acute inferior infarction. Anatomically, it is located at the level of the AV node, accounting for the fact that QRS duration tends to be normal. The junctional pacemaker is usually reliable, and observation of the patient until the conduction disturbance resolves is often all that is needed.

In contrast, *Mobitz II second-degree AV block*

Lead MCL₁

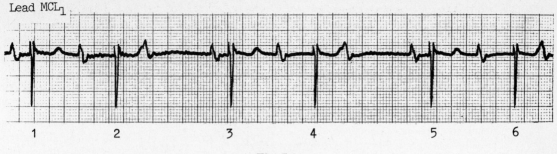

Fig. 7-6

Lead MCL₁

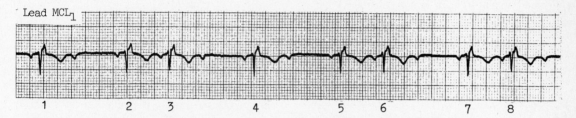

Fig. 7-7. From Grauer, K.: Am. Fam. Physician **28**:162, 1983.

Lead II

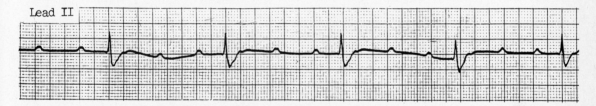

Fig. 7-8

is more often associated with anteroseptal infarction. It is much less common than Mobitz I and occurs at a lower anatomic level in the conduction system (it is always subnodal). As a result, the QRS complex is usually wide, and the escape focus is less reliable. There is a strong tendency for Mobitz II second-degree AV block to develop into complete AV block, often with little warning. Consequently, its detection in the setting of acute infarction should prompt immediate pacemaker insertion.

Electrocardiographically, Mobitz II second-degree AV block is recognized by nonconduction of one or more beats despite the maintenance of a constant PR interval. The atrial rate remains regular throughout (Fig. 7-7). These characteristics of Mobitz I and II second-degree AV blocks are summarized in Table 7-1.

PROBLEM: Consider the rhythm strips shown in Figs. 7-8 and 7-9. How would you classify the types of AV conduction disturbances that they represent?

Table 7-1. Comparison of Mobitz I and II AV blocks

	Mobitz I	Mobitz II
Clinical occurrence	Usually associated with inferior myocardial infarction Relatively frequent Usually transient	Usually associated with anteroseptal myocardial infarction Uncommon Often progresses to complete heart block
Anatomic level	At the AV node	Below the AV node
ECG characteristics	Gradually lengthening PR interval until a beat is dropped: First-degree AV block is common QRS complex is usually narrow	Constant PR interval until one or more beats are dropped: PR interval is usually normal QRS complex is usually wide
Treatment	Observation usually suffices, provided that ventricular response is adequate	Pacemaker insertion is required

ANSWER TO FIG. 7-8: The atrial rate is regular at 115 beats/min in Fig. 7-8. The ventricular rate is also regular at just under 40 beats/min; however, each QRS complex is preceded by a P wave with a fixed PR interval. Thus this cannot be complete AV block but must instead be a form of *second degree AV block*. The rhythm in Fig. 7-8 is referred to as *high-grade* (or *high-degree*) *heart block*, since only one out of every three atrial beats is conducted to the ventricles. (The QRS complex is wide, suggesting that the anatomic level of the block is low down in the conduction system.)

• • •

PROBLEM: Examine Fig. 7-9. The atrial rate in Fig. 7-9 is regular at 58 beats/min. The ventricular rate is also regular at 29 beats/min. Each QRS complex is preceded by P wave with a constant PR interval, but only half of the atrial impulses are conducted to the ventricles. Does the rhythm in Fig. 7-9 represent Mobitz I or Mobitz II second-degree AV block?

ANSWER TO FIG. 7-9: By definition, Fig. 7-9 is *second-degree AV block with 2:1 AV conduction*, since every other atrial impulse is blocked. Theoretically, this could be *either* Mobitz I or Mobitz II second-degree AV block. Granted, a constant PR interval precedes every QRS complex and suggests Mobitz II, but since only one QRS complex at a time is conducted, the opportunity for the PR interval to lengthen before dropping a beat does not exist.

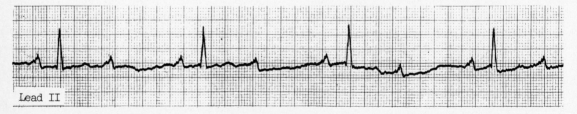

Lead II

Fig. 7-9

The two following factors suggest that this rhythm is more likely to be Mobitz I: the normal duration of the QRS complex and the presence of first-degree AV block. Both of these features are more commonly seen with Mobitz I (Table 7-1), but *one cannot absolutely distinguish between Mobitz I and Mobitz II second-degree AV block in the presence of 2:1 AV conduction.*

PROBLEM: This patient was medicated with 0.5 mg atropine, and shortly thereafter the rhythm shown in Fig. 7-10 was observed. What has happened?

ANSWER TO FIG. 7-10: Second-degree AV block is no longer present in Fig. 7-10. The rhythm is now *sinus bradycardia* with *first-degree AV block*. This strengthens the case that Fig. 7-9 represented Mobitz I second-degree AV block, since Mobitz II would be much less likely to respond so easily to medical treatment.

Even when more than one QRS complex is

conducted before the dropped beat, the diagnosis of Wenckebach block is not always as obvious as in Fig. 7-6. In Fig. 7-11 a long Wenckebach cycle begins with beat 3 and continues until a beat is finally dropped after QRS complex 12. If one merely compared consecutive PR intervals during the middle of this run, it would not be at all apparent that the PR interval was progressively lengthening. Only by comparing the last PR interval just before the dropped beat (the PR interval of beat 12) with the first PR interval in the run (the PR interval of beat 3) can this relationship be established. With the onset of the next Wenckebach cycle (beat 13), the PR interval has again shortened.

Another characteristic of Wenckebach blocks is observed here. *The pause containing the dropped beat* (the R-R interval between beats 12 and 13) *is less than twice the shortest R-R interval.* This is a helpful feature to look for in differentiating Wenckebach blocks from Mobitz II second-degree AV block, in which the pause is precisely twice the regular R-R interval, and

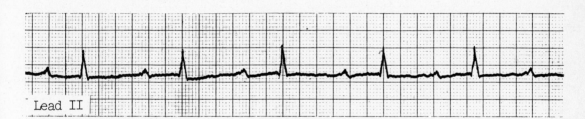

Fig. 7-10

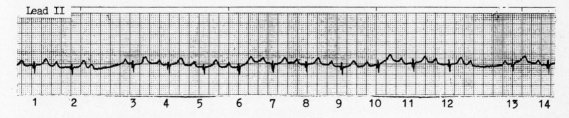

Fig. 7-11

from sinus pauses, in which the interval, including the dropped beat, is often more than twice the regular R-R interval.

GROUP BEATING

A final feature to look for in diagnosing Wenckebach blocks is *group beating*. This produces a *regular irregularity* in the rhythm. Group beating is well illustrated in Fig. 7-12 in which two groups of three beats each (beats 1-3 and 4-6) and two groups of two beats each (7-8 and 9-10) are evident. Inspection of the PR intervals for this rhythm strip reveals the progressively lengthening PR interval in each group until a beat is dropped. Thus Fig. 7-12 represents Wenckebach second-degree AV block with 4:3 and 3:2 AV conduction.

A number of dysrhythmias in addition to Mobitz I second-degree AV block may exhibit Wenckebach-type conduction disturbances. These include SA Wenckebach (of both the Mobitz I and Mobitz II varieties), Wenckebach conduction in the presence of atrial fibrillation or atrial flutter, and AV nodal rhythm with retrograde Wenckebach conduction. Although the mechanism of these arrhythmias is beyond the scope of this text, recognition of group beating may arouse suspicion of its presence.

PROBLEM: For example, determine the mechanism of the dysrhythmia shown in Fig. 7-13.

ANSWER TO FIG. 7-13: P waves are seen to march through the rhythm strip although at a somewhat irregular rate (Fig. 7-13). There is a *regular irregularity* to the ventricular rhythm (i.e., three *groups* of *short-long cycles* are seen). The trick lies with beats 1, 3, and 5. On close inspection the QRS configuration of these beats can be seen to differ slightly from that of beats 2, 4, and 6. Moreover, the PR interval of beat 5 is definitely too short to conduct, implying that this beat and the two oth-

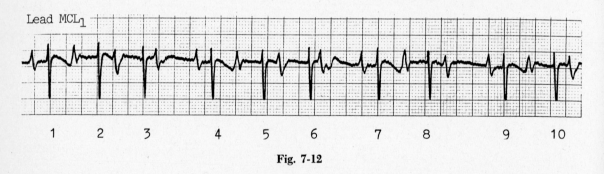

Fig. 7-12

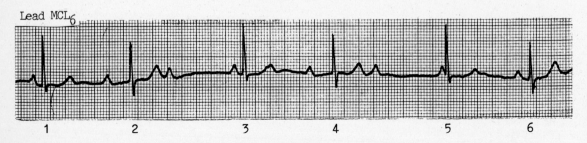

Fig. 7-13

ers like it (beats 1 and 3) are junctional escape beats.

The important point of this rather difficult rhythm strip is that the presence of dropped beats and group beating should incite one to consider the possibility of some type of Wenckebach conduction. (Third-degree AV block is unlikely because of the irregularity of the ventricular response.)

• • •

PROBLEM: A last point on group beating is that this phenomenon does *not* always represent Wenckebach block. Can you determine why the regular irregularity of the rhythm shown in Fig. 7-14 is *not* the result of Mobitz I second-degree AV block?

ANSWER TO FIG. 7-14: Group beating is evident in Fig. 7-14, but close inspection of the T waves following beats 2, 5, and 8 reveals an extra peak that is not present in the T waves of the other beats. This extra peak is caused by the presence of a premature P wave that occurs every fourth beat. Because these PACs occur early in the refractory period, they are blocked. The rhythm is therefore *atrial quadrigeminy* with *blocked PACs*.

Fig. 7-15 is taken from the same patient a short time later and again demonstrates frequent PACs. The PAC that peaks the T wave following beat 6 is blocked, but those following beats 3, 7, and 8 are conducted with different degrees of aberrancy. *The commonest cause of a pause is a blocked PAC!*

CLINICAL SIGNIFICANCE AND TREATMENT OF AV BLOCKS

A firm appreciation of the various types of AV blocks and the ability to separate those dysrhythmias that mimic them are essential skills for anyone involved in cardiac resuscitation. Treatment and prognosis depend on accurate diagnosis of the degree of AV conduction disturbance. Survival of patients with first-degree AV block and Mobitz I second-degree AV block is generally not jeopardized by the conduction disturbance itself so that no treatment other than observation is usually needed. In contrast, pacemaker insertion is recommended for patients with Mobitz II second-degree AV block.

The situation with third-degree (complete)

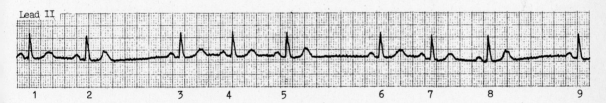

Fig. 7-14

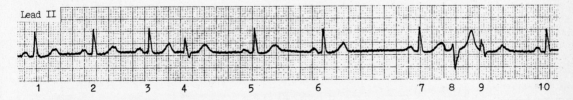

Fig. 7-15

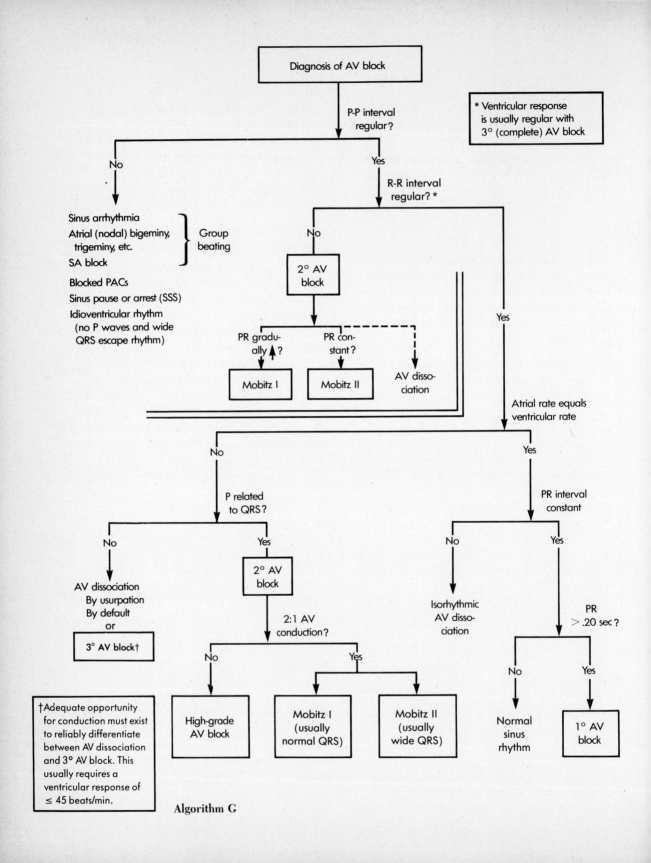

Diagnosis of AV block

P-P interval regular?

* Ventricular response is usually regular with 3° (complete) AV block

No

Yes

R-R interval regular? *

Sinus arrhythmia
Atrial (nodal) bigeminy, trigeminy, etc.
SA block
} Group beating

Blocked PACs
Sinus pause or arrest (SSS)
Idioventricular rhythm (no P waves and wide QRS escape rhythm)

No

2° AV block

Yes

PR gradually ↑?

PR constant?

AV dissociation

Mobitz I

Mobitz II

Atrial rate equals ventricular rate

No

Yes

P related to QRS?

PR interval constant

No

Yes

No

Yes

AV dissociation
By usurpation
By default
or

3° AV block†

2° AV block

Isorhythmic AV dissociation

PR > .20 sec?

2:1 AV conduction?

No

Yes

No

Yes

†Adequate opportunity for conduction must exist to reliably differentiate between AV dissociation and 3° AV block. This usually requires a ventricular response of ≤ 45 beats/min.

High-grade AV block

Mobitz I (usually normal QRS)

Mobitz II (usually wide QRS)

Normal sinus rhythm

1° AV block

Algorithm G

Table 7-2. Clinical significance of third-degree AV block

		Inferior infarction	
	Anterior infarction	Junctional escape focus (narrow QRS complex)	Idioventricular escape focus (wide QRS complex)
Rate of ventricular response	30-60 beats/min (depending on site of escape focus)	40-60 beats/min	30-40 beats/min
Usual duration of conduction disturbance	Long-term	Transient	Long-term
Response to atropine	Poor	Good	Poor
Recommended treatment	Pacemaker insertion	Observation if hemodynamically stable Treat syptomatic bradycardia and/or hypotension with 1. Atropine 2. Dopamine, epinephrine, or isoproterenol infusion 3. Pacemaker insertion	Pacemaker insertion

AV block is somewhat more complicated. Pacemaker insertion is routinely performed in patients who develop complete AV block as the result of acute anterior infarction. The escape pacemaker tends to be idioventricular (wide QRS complex) and is often associated with a slow heart rate and hemodynamic compromise. On the other hand, complete AV block that develops with acute inferior infarction may occur with a stable junctional escape rhythm (narrow QRS complex) that is able to keep the patient hemodynamically compensated. The mechanism of AV block in this setting may simply reflect increased parasympathetic tone and/or ischemia of the AV node rather than irreversible myocardial damage. The conduction defect is usually transient. If the heart rate remains close to 60 beats/min, no treatment at all may be indicated.

With slower heart rates, atropine may effectively accelerate the ventricular response and/or improve AV conduction. Pacemaker insertion is often not needed (Table 7-2).

Review of Fig. 7-9 brings to light an important exception to these generalities. Despite the fact that this rhythm more than likely represents Mobitz I second-degree AV block (usually a benign disorder), the ventricular response is clearly inadequate. If the patient were not to respond to medical therapy, pacemaker insertion would be essential. If one compares the degree of hemodynamic compromise of a patient with the rhythm in Fig. 7-9 to one with third-degree (complete) AV block and a junctional escape rhythm at 60 beats/min), the former patient (with Mobitz I second-degree AV block and a ventricular response of 29 beats/min) has

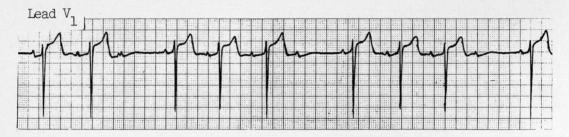

Lead V_1

Fig. 7-16. From Grauer, K.: Am. Fam. Physician **28**:162, 1983.

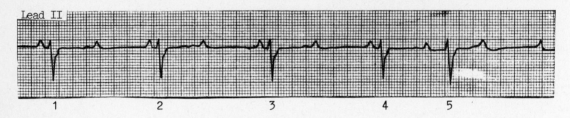

Lead II

1 2 3 4 5

Fig. 7-17

the more clinically significant conduction disturbance. Thus more than just the degree of AV block, *the ventricular response becomes a critical determinant of the clinical impact of the conduction disturbance on an individual patient*.

PROBLEM: As a review of the material covered in this chapter, interpret the nine dysrhythmias shown in Figs. 7-16 to 7-24. (Note: Some masqueraders of AV block have been included to keep you honest.)

ANSWER TO FIG. 7-16: The atrial rate is regular at 75 beats/min in Fig. 7-16. The QRS complex is of normal duration. Group beating is evident with a progressively lengthening PR interval in each group until a beat is dropped. This is *second-degree AV block, Mobitz I* with 3:2 and 4:3 AV conduction.

ANSWER TO FIG. 7-17: The atrial rate in Fig. 7-17 is regular at 75 beats/min. The QRS complex appears to be slightly prolonged, although it is hard to be certain of where the QRS complex ends and the ST segment

begins. There is 2:1 AV conduction early in the rhythm strip in which the PR interval remains constant for beats 1 to 4. It would be difficult to differentiate between Mobitz I and Mobitz II second-degree AV blocks if the rhythm strip ended here. However, the PR interval of beat 5 lengthens with respect to the PR of beat 4, the telltale sign of Wenckebach. Since it would be unlikely for a patient to switch abruptly from Mobitz I to Mobitz II second-degree AV block, the entire rhythm strip probably represents Wenckebach with 2:1 and 3:2 AV conduction.

ANSWER TO FIG. 7-18: One is struck by the phenomenon of group beating. However, examination of the P-P interval reveals that the P waves following beats 2 and 6 occur early in Fig. 7-18. These are PACs in which conduction to the ventricles is blocked because of their marked prematurity. Thus no AV block is present, and the pauses are the result of blocked PACs. (*The commonest cause of a pause is a blocked PAC.*)

Lead V_1

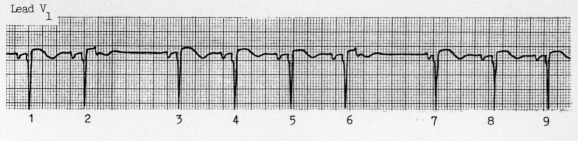

1   2   3   4   5   6   7   8   9

Fig. 7-18

Lead II

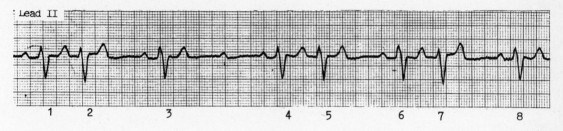

1   2   3   4   5   6   7   8

Fig. 7-19

The PR interval of beat 7 is significantly shorter than the PR interval of the other normally conducted beats in this tracing. This PR interval is too short to represent normal sinus conduction. Thus beat 7 must be a junctional escape beat that arose before the normal sinus impulse could be conducted to the ventricles.

ANSWER TO FIG. 7-19: Fig. 7-19 is difficult, since at first glance no P waves can be seen in front of beats 2, 5, and 7. Two P waves in a row occur before beat 4. If one uses this P-P interval and walks out the atrial rate, the missing P waves are seen to coincide with the T waves preceding beats 2, 5, and 7. Thus several beats are dropped and a type of second-degree AV block is present. Since the QRS complex is widened and each QRS complex is preceded by a P wave with a fixed PR interval, this probably represents Mobitz II second-degree AV block. Additional support for this diagnosis comes from the fact that two beats in a row are dropped during the longest pause.

ANSWER TO FIG. 7-20: The atrial rate is regular at 130 beats/min in Fig. 7-20. The QRS complex is wide and regular at 45 beats/min. The PR interval is constantly changing as "P waves march through the QRS complex." This is *third-degree AV block*.

ANSWER TO FIG. 7-21: Although group beating is simulated in Fig. 7-21, inspection for atrial activity reveals marked variation in the P-P interval. Since each QRS complex is preceded by a normal-appearing P wave with a constant PR interval, sinus conduction is present. This is *sinus arrhythmia*.

ANSWER TO FIG. 7-22: The rhythm is irregularly irregular in Fig. 7-22. Small upright deflections simulating P waves are noted between each R-R interval, but these appear to be related to the QRS complex that precedes them rather than to the subsequent QRS complex (the R-"P" interval is fixed). The ventricular response is too irregular for this to be a junctional rhythm with a retrograde P wave.

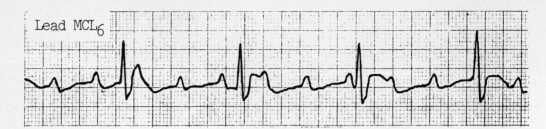

Fig. 7-20

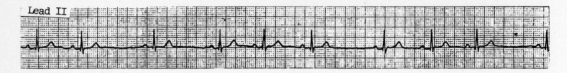

Fig. 7-21

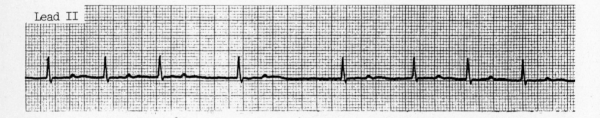

Fig. 7-22

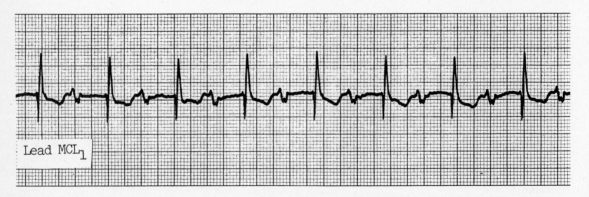

Fig. 7-23

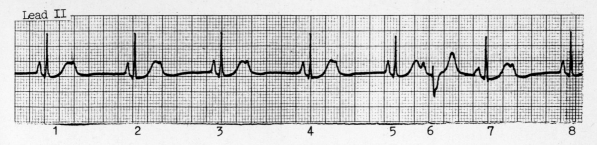

Fig. 7-24

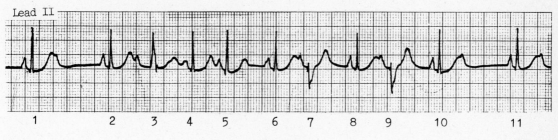

Fig. 7-25

This is *atrial fibrillation* with a controlled ventricular response. The small upright deflections are T waves.

ANSWER TO FIG. 7-23: In Fig. 7-23 the rhythm is regular at 70 beats/min. Again the problem is deciding whether the P waves are related to the preceding or subsequent QRS complexes. The latter is more likely, making this *sinus rhythm* with *first-degree AV block*. An RBBB configuration is present in this right-sided lead.

ANSWER TO FIG. 7-24: Sinus bradycardia at 50 beats/min is simulated in Fig. 7-24 for the first five beats until interrupted by an aberrantly conducted PAC (beat 6). However, close inspection of all the T waves in this rhythm strip reveals that they are notched. The actual rhythm is *atrial bigeminy with blocked PACs*.

A short time later the rhythm strip shown in Fig. 7-25 is taken from the same patient. The underlying rhythm is still atrial bigeminy. PACs are conducted almost normally for beats 3 and 5 and with aberration for beats 7 and 9, whereas the PACs that notch the T waves of beats 1 and 10 are blocked.

SUGGESTED READINGS

American Heart Association Subcommittee on Emergency Cardiac Care: Standards and guidelines for cardiopulmonary resuscitation (CPR) and emergency cardiac care (ECC), JAMA 244:453-509, 1980.

Marriott, H.J.L., and Conover, M.H.B.: Advanced concepts in arrhythmias, St. Louis, 1983, The C.V. Mosby Co. pp. 268-290.

Morelli, R.L.: The temporary cardiac pacemaker. In Auerbach, P.S., and Budassi, S.A., (editors: Cardiac arrest and CPR, Rockville, Md., 1983, Aspen Systems Corp., pp. 77-117.

PART THREE

PROBLEM SOLVING IN CARDIAC ARREST

CHAPTER 8

Case studies

CASE STUDY 1

You are working in the emergency department where a patient collapses. He cannot be aroused. A *code blue* is called, and a full complement of qualified assistants assemble around you waiting for your next command. How would you proceed?

ANALYSIS
1. Confirm unresponsiveness.
2. Open the airway.
3. Verify apnea.
4. Verfiy pulselessness.

5. Give four full breaths, and begin CPR. (There is no need to call for help, since you are surrounded by qualified assistants. They may be instructed to carry on CPR for you.)
6. Bring over the crash cart, turn on the defibrillator, and apply the quick-look paddles.

All of these steps are accomplished within 40 seconds, and you observe the rhythm shown in Fig. 8-1. What is this rhythm? How would you treat it?

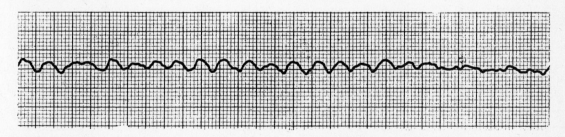

Fig. 8-1

ANALYSIS OF FIG. 8-1: There is a total lack of organized electrical activity; the rhythm is *ventricular fibrillation*.

7. Apply conductive medium to the paddles, assure that no one is in contact with the patient, apply firm pressure to the paddles (pressing down with approximately 25 pounds of force), and *defibrillate* the patient with *200 J of delivered energy*.

The patient remains pulseless and unresponsive. Reapplication of the quick-look paddles reveals the rhythm shown in Fig. 8-2. What would you do now?

ANALYSIS OF FIG. 8-2: The patient is still in ventricular fibrillation.

8. *Repeat defibrillation* at the same 200 J energy level as soon as possible. (Minimiz-

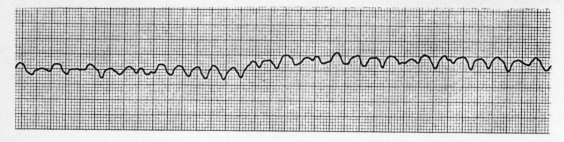

Fig. 8-2

ing the time between these two electrical discharges is important, since rapid succession of countershocks has been shown to decrease transthoracic resistance and facilitate electrical conversion by the second countershock.)

The patient remains pulseless and in ventricular fibrillation. What should be done next?

ANALYSIS

9. *Resume CPR.*
10. *Establish an airway* and *intubate* the patient if possible. Intubation is *not* recommended before the initial two defibrillation attempts, since it consumes valuable time and requires the cessation of CPR. Success at defibrillation is inversely proportional to the amount of time between the onset of ventricular fibrillation and the application of electrical countershock. (Intubation may occasionally not even be needed if defibrillation successfully restores an effective cardiac rhythm.)
11. *Establish intravenous access.*
12. Administer 1 mg of *epinephrine* by either the intravenous or intratracheal route. Follow this with *sodium bicarbonate* "as appropriate."

Administration of cardiac drugs for ventricular fibrillation is *not* recommended before the initial two countershocks if a defibrillator is available, since this would only delay the application of electrical countershock.

Sodium bicarbonate is dispensed in 50 ml prefilled syringes that contain 50 mEq of drug. "Appropriate dosing" depends greatly on the amount of time that transpires from the onset of the cardiac arrest. When the period of arrest is brief (such as in this case study), no bicarbonate is indicated. The resuscitative efforts were promptly undertaken, and there probably has not been sufficient time for metabolic acidosis to develop. When the period of arrest is longer, an initial dose of 1 mEq of sodium bicarbonate per kilogram of body weight (usually 1 to 1½ ampules) is recommended. Two ampules are sometimes given at the onset when 3 to 5 minutes have elapsed from the time that cardiovascular collapse occurs.

Additional boluses of sodium bicarbonate are ideally governed by the results of ABG determinations. Iatrogenic metabolic alkalosis from the overzealous administration of sodium bicarbonate is difficult to reverse and may lead to seizures and even the death of the patient. Consequently, ABGs should be obtained at the earliest opportunity. If ABGs are not available (as they would not be during transport of the patient in cardiac arrest to the hospital), one may empirically repeat one half of the initial dose every 10 to 15 minutes while CPR is in progress.

Epinephrine is dispensed in 10 ml prefilled syringes that contain 1 mg of epinephrine in a 1:10,000 dilution. The drug may be given intravenously, intratracheally, or by intracardiac injection. Excellent absorption and rapid onset of action is achieved following administration of epinephrine by either the intravenous or intratracheal route. The intracardiac route, on the other hand, is no longer recommended except as a last resort. Intracardiac injection of epinephrine interrupts CPR and has been associated with a number of severe complications including laceration of a coronary artery, pericardial tamponade, intramyocardial injection of drug with resultant intractable ventricular fibrillation, and pneumothorax.

In the past, administration of epinephrine was recommended only after giving sodium bicarbonate. Although catecholamines may work better once acidosis has been corrected, two practical points argue for choosing epinephrine as the first pharmacologic agent administered during cardiac arrest:

• Sodium bicarbonate is dispensed in ampules of a much larger volume that require more time to infuse.

• The intravenous line must be thoroughly flushed before giving epinephrine if sodium bicarbonate was just recently infused, since catecholamines are partially inactivated by an alkaline solution.

If both intratracheal and intravenous access are established, drug delivery may be optimized by the simultaneous administration of epinephrine intratracheally and sodium bicarbonate intravenously.

One milligram of epinephrine is given intravenously. The respiratory therapist draws a set of ABGs from the femoral pulse that is palpated with external chest compressions. What should you do at this point?

ANALYSIS
13. Have your assistants hook up monitoring leads or preferably an ECG machine to the patient.
14. Recheck the patient for responsiveness, the presence of a pulse, and a rhythm on the ECG.

The patient remains pulseless and unresponsive. The rhythm is shown in Fig. 8-3. What is there to do now?

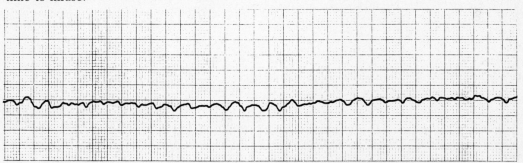

Fig. 8-3

ANALYSIS OF FIG. 8-3
15. The patient should again be defibrillated, since he is still in ventricular fibrillation. This third time the maximum delivered energy level should be used (usually 360 J).

Defibrillation produces the rhythm shown in Fig. 8-4. How should you proceed?

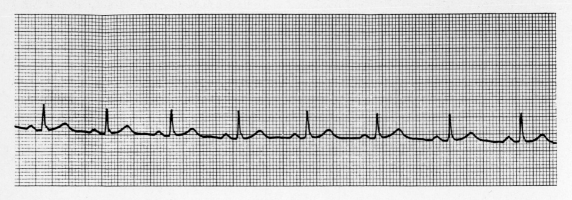

Fig. 8-4

ANALYSIS OF FIG. 8-4

16. *Check for a pulse!*

No one can feel a pulse. The patient remains unresponsive and is cyanotic. What is the rhythm that is shown in Fig. 8-4? How should this patient be treated?

ANALYSIS: The rhythm in Fig. 8-4 is sinus. *EMD* is present, since there is organized electrical activity (the monitor shows normal-appearing sinus-initiated complexes) without any evidence of effective myocardial contraction (pulselessness). Treatment is similar to that recommended for asystole.

17. Resume CPR.
18. Administer epinephrine and sodium bicarbonate as appropriate. (The ABGs drawn by the respiratory therapist will be ready momentarily.)
19. Consider the use of calcium chloride.
20. Search for a potentially reversible cause of EMD such as inadequate ventilation (intubation of the right mainstem bronchus, tension pneumothorax), pericardial effusion with tamponade, persistent acidosis or other metabolic derangement, or hypovolemia (cardiogenic shock, dehydration, acute blood loss).

Auscultation of the chest reveals the absence of breath sounds on the left. Withdrawal of the endotracheal tube by about an inch results in the return of equal bilateral breath sounds. Shortly thereafter a strong pulse can be felt, and a blood pressure of 95/70 mm Hg is obtained. The monitor continues to show sinus rhythm.

21. Administer a 50 to 100 mg bolus of *lidocaine*. Follow this with an IV infusion made by mixing 2 g of lidocaine in 500 ml of D_5W, and set it to run at 30 drops/min (2 mg/min).
22. Transfer the patient to the coronary care unit.

Discussion

This case illustrates a reasonable protocol to follow for resuscitating the patient found in ventricular fibrillation. Several points deserve special mention.

Notable for its absence is the precordial thump. The effectiveness of this maneuver has never been convincingly demonstrated, and reports of asystole have occasionally followed its use. At present the precordial thump is only recommended for ventricular tachycardia or ventricular fibrillation that occurs while the patient is being directly observed and monitored electrocardiographically by trained personnel. Use of the precordial thump was not indicated in this case study even though the patient's collapse was witnessed, since he was not being monitored at the time.

It is important to emphasize that the likelihood of successfully resuscitating a patient in cardiac arrest is inversely proportional to the interval between the onset of ventricular fibrillation and the application of countershock. Thus *all patients should be defibrillated as soon as the diagnosis of ventricular fibrillation has been established.* Delay for the purpose of intubation and/or starting an IV line to administer epinephrine or sodium bicarbonate is unwarranted and may adversely affect the chances for survival. This recommendation represents a change from previously suggested guidelines. In the past an initial 2-minute period of CPR was allowed during which drugs could be administered and circulated, and the patient could be intubated. This new protocol applies both to patients with cardiac arrest in the emergency department or in the field; as soon as ventricular fibrillation has been documented, the patient should be defibrillated with 200 J of delivered energy.

If the initial two attempts at defibrillation are unsuccessful, it is then reasonable to intubate the patient, establish intravenous access, and administer epinephrine and sodium bicarbonate as appropriate. If ventricular fibrillation persists, a third attempt at defibrillation should be tried.

The energy levels recommended for defibrillation have also changed. Initial defibrillation with as little as 175 J of delivered energy has been shown to be as effective in converting ventricular fibrillation as countershock with 320 J, yet it is associated with a lower incidence of advanced AV block after defibrillation. Consequently, the delivered energy of the two initial countershock attempts should probably be limited to 200 J. If this is unsuccessful, the third attempt should be with the maximum delivered energy (usually 360 J).

What would you have done if the patient in this case study had remained in ventricular fibrillation following the third countershock?

ANALYSIS

23. *Look for reasons to explain the refractory ventricular fibrillation.* Was the Airway secure? Was mechanical Breathing effective? (Were good bilateral breath sounds present? Was the PaO_2 adequate?) Was Circulation reestablished? (Did CPR produce a pulse?) Was the patient still acidotic? These are some of the potentially reversible factors that might account for refractory ventricular fibrillation. Alternatively, the patient may have suffered a massive myocardial infarction or ruptured an aortic aneurysm, factors that would be extremely difficult to reverse at this point by any therapy.

24. Consider pharmacologic treatment for refractory ventricular fibrillation.
    A. Lidocaine.
    B. *Bretylium tosylate.* Studies have suggested that bretylium may stabilize the myocardium of patients with refractory ventricular fibrillation in a manner that facilitates conversion to sinus rhythm with subsequent countershock. Although controlled studies in this setting are difficult to come by, bretylium may be the drug of choice for patients with refractory ventricular fibrillation.

For ventricular fibrillation *bretylium* should be administered IV as a bolus of 5 to 10 mg/kg (usually about 1 ampule or 500 mg) and infused over a 2-minute period. This dose may be repeated if needed in 15 to 30 minutes up to a maximum total dose of 30 mg/kg. The onset of action of bretylium may be delayed for up to 15 minutes. Thus the resuscitation effort *must* be continued for an appropriate period of time once the decision has been made to use the drug.

Bretylium rarely effects spontaneous conversion to sinus rhythm from ventricular fibrillation but rather facilitates conversion with subsequent countershock. Prevention of recurrence may then be accomplished by initiation of a bretylium infusion. (Mix 2 g in 500 ml of D_5W, and set the drip to run in at 1 to 2 mg/min). Alternatively, a lidocaine infusion may be used to prevent recurrence once the patient has been converted out of ventricular fibrillation.

Bretylium is also an effective agent for treating ventricular tachycardia that has been resistant to standard therapy. One ampule (500 mg) is diluted in 50 ml of D_5W and infused over a 10-minute period.

The actions of bretylium are complex and include an initial release of catecholamines, which may initially cause hypertension, followed by a postganglionic adrenergic blocking effect. This latter action may result in hypotension, which is the most common side effect of the drug.

At the present time bretylium is recommended for the treatment of refractory ventricular fibrillation and/or refractory ventricular tachycardia. It should *not* be used as a first-line agent for PVCs, which are better treated with lidocaine.

If the patient in this case study remained in ventricular fibrillation after administering the initial dose of bretylium and applying countershock, the treatment cycle should be repeated. This would entail the additional use of epinephrine and sodium bicarbonate as appropriate, a second (and possibly a third) dose of bretylium, and further attempts at defibrillation until the patient was either converted out of ventricular fibrillation or cardiovascular unresponsiveness could be conclusively established.

CASE STUDY 2

A 50-year-old man develops chest pain at a restaurant. He is promptly attended to by the mobile EMS unit who prepare him for transport to the emergency department. They contact you and report that the patient is diaphoretic and still complaining of severe chest pain. His pulse is irregular, blood pressure is 100/70 mm Hg, and telemetry rhythm is shown in Fig. 8-5. What should you have the EMS unit do at this point?

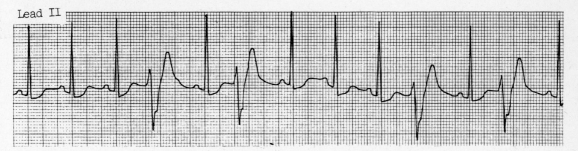

Fig. 8-5

ANALYSIS OF FIG. 8-5: The rhythm is sinus at 95 beats/min, and frequent *PVCs* are present. With chest pain suggestive of possible acute myocardial infarction, PVCs need to be treated.

1. Administer 4 to 6 L/min of *oxygen* by nasal cannula.
2. Establish an IV line.
3. Administer *morphine sulfate*, 3 to 5 mg IV repeated every 3 to 5 minutes as needed for relief of pain.

4. Administer a 75 to 100 mg bolus of *lidocaine* (1 mg/kg of body weight). Mix 2 g in 500 ml of D_5W, and begin a lidocaine infusion to run at 30 drops/min (2 mg/min).

The patient's chest pain markedly decreases with 5 mg of IV morphine and the use of supplemental oxygen. Rhythm strips taken en route to the emergency department 5 and 10 minutes following administration of the lidocaine bolus are shown in Figs. 8-6 and 8-7. What is your interpretation? How would you advise the EMS unit at this point?

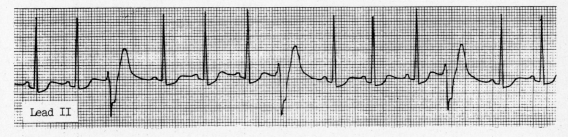

Fig. 8-6

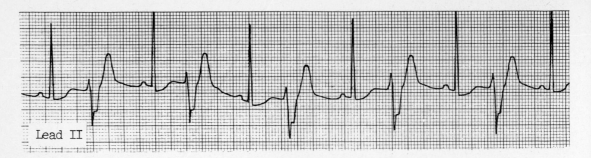

Fig. 8-7

ANALYSIS OF FIGS. 8-6 AND 8-7: The underlying rhythm is still sinus, but frequent PVCs persist. As before, these PVCs are *unifocal* (they all have a similar configuration) and manifest a *fixed coupling interval* (they are all about 0.44 second from the preceding QRS complex). Fig. 8-6 demonstrates *ventricular quadrigeminy* (every fourth beat is a PVC) and Fig. 8-7 shows *ventricular bigeminy* (every other beat is a PVC).

5. Give the patient another 50 to 75 mg bolus of lidocaine. Increasing the drip to a rate of 3 mg/min may be considered but is *not* essential (see pp. 43-45).

Since the half-life of lidocaine in its central compartment is only about 10 minutes, a decision as to whether or not additional boluses are needed must be made at this point. The persistence of frequent PVCs indicates the need for a second bolus.

Minutes later the ambulance arrives in the emergency department. The patient is now comfortable, and the paramedics triumphantly hand you the rhythm strip shown in Fig. 8-8, taken shortly after the second bolus of lidocaine was given. What do you see?

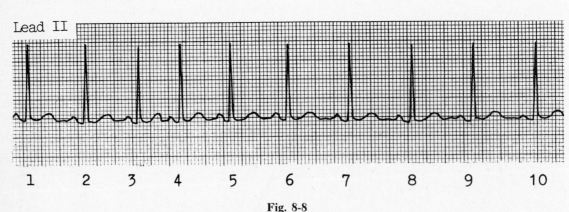

Fig. 8-8

ANALYSIS OF FIG. 8-8: Normal sinus rhythm is reestablished with the exception of beat 4, which is premature. As opposed to the PVCs present in Figs. 8-5 to 8-7, in which the premature beats are wide and bizarre in shape, a

P wave precedes beat 4 in Fig. 8-8, and the QRS configuration of this beat is virtually identical to that of the other sinus conducted beats. This is a *PAC*. Whereas PVCs with acute ischemia may predispose the patient to the development of ventricular fibrillation and should be suppressed with lidocaine, PACs in general do not need to be treated.

In the emergency department the patient is switched to a right-sided monitoring lead system (i.e., an MCL_1 lead). Telemetry continues to show sinus rhythm. A 12-lead ECG is done and suggests acute anterior infarction. Arrange-ments are made for transfer to the coronary care unit, but before this can be accomplished the nurse hands you the rhythm strip shown in Fig. 8-9. The patient is still comfortable at this point and is maintaining a blood pressure of 100/70 mm Hg. He shows no signs of congestive heart failure. What do you see in Fig. 8-9? Would you administer more lidocaine?

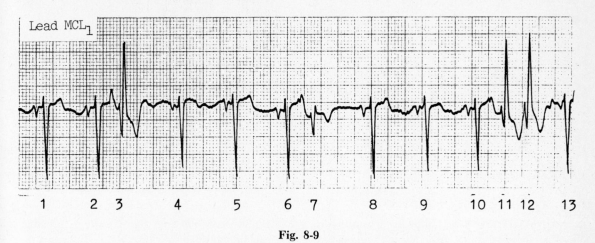

Lead MCL_1

Fig. 8-9

ANALYSIS OF FIG. 8-9: The rhythm is sinus at about 90 beats/min. The QRS configuration of beats 3, 7, 11, and 12 differs from that of the normal sinus beats, raising the question as to whether these are PVCs or PACs that are conducted aberrantly? Answering this question is more than an academic exercise because PVCs might require additional treatment, whereas PACs in a patient who is otherwise comfortable could probably be safely observed.

The three most helpful features to look for in recognizing aberrantly conducted PACs and differentiating them from PVCs are the following:
- *Similar initial deflection* of the anomalous beats to the normal sinus beats.
- *RBBB configuration* (i.e., rSR') in a right-sided monitoring lead.
- *Premature P wave*, which often deforms the preceding T wave.

All three of these features can be identified for the beats in question in Fig. 8-9. Specifically, all of these abnormal-appearing complexes begin with an initial upward deflection as do the normally conducted beats. A complete RBBB pattern is evident for beats 3, 11, and 12, and an incomplete RBBB pattern for beat 7 is present. Finally, careful inspection reveals that a premature P wave precedes each of these beats, peaking the T wave of beat 2 and notching the T waves of beats 6 and 10.

Additional supportive evidence favoring aberrancy over ventricular ectopy includes the absence of a full compensatory pause and the fact that the abnormal QRS complexes, although wider than the normally conducted beats, are only 0.11 second in duration. (The interval containing a PVC often demonstrates a full compensatory pause, and the QRS duration of a PVC usually exceeds 0.11 second). Taken together these factors overwhelmingly favor aberrancy.

What would you have done if instead of the aberrantly conducted beats shown in Fig. 8-9, the patient was having runs of anomalous complexes similar to those of beats 7 to 12 in Fig. 8-10?

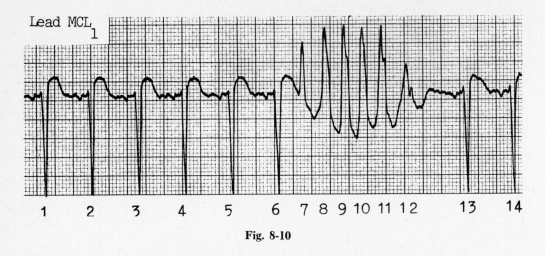

Fig. 8-10

ANALYSIS OF FIG. 8-10: Following six sinus conducted beats, the QRS complex widens and takes on a different appearance. The presence of a monophasic R-wave configuration in this right-sided monitoring lead strongly suggests that beats 7 to 12 represent a run of ventricular tachycardia. Sinus rhythm resumes with beat 13 after a postectopic pause.

6. Consider giving a third bolus of lidocaine.

or

7. Begin *procainamide*. Increments of 100 mg can be administered intravenously over a 5-minute period until either the dysrhythmia is controlled, a total loading dose of 1 g is given, or untoward side effects appear (hypotension or widening of the QRS complex). This may be followed by a continuous procainamide infusion at a rate of 1 to 4 mg/min.

Should these runs of ventricular tachycardia fail to be controlled with procainamide, one might consider a trial of *bretylium*.

CASE STUDY 3

A 65-year-old woman came to the emergency department complaining of a "fluttering" in her chest that developed within the past hour. She was not in any distress, did not complain of chest pain and had a blood pressure of 90/60 mm Hg at the time the rhythm strip shown in Fig. 8-11 was recorded. How would you interpret this tracing? What would you do at this point?

ANALYSIS OF FIG. 8-11: A regular tachydysrhythmia at a rate of about 150 beats/min is present. Although definite P waves are not seen, this rhythm was assumed to be supraventricular because the patient was awake, was alert, and had a reasonable blood pressure.

The patient was given 5 mg of valium orally for sedation and an IV line was started. A 12-lead ECG (Fig. 8-12) was obtained and interpreted as

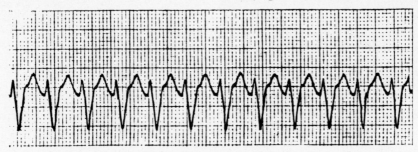

Fig. 8-11

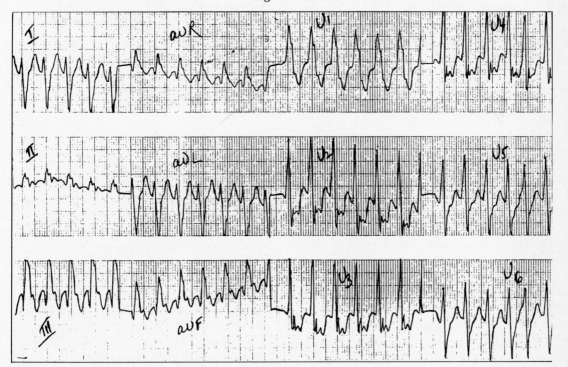

Fig. 8-12

showing SVT with RBBB and posterior hemiblock. Do you agree with the assessment and management of this patient so far?

The fluttering sensation continued, but the patient's blood pressure remained stable, and she was not really uncomfortable. Thirty minutes later someone informs you that the patient's basic rhythm has changed (Fig. 8-13). What has happened? Retrospectively, how would you interpret Figs. 8-11 and 8-12? What would have been a more optimal plan of management for this patient?

ANALYSIS OF FIG. 8-13: Sinus tachycardia is present in Fig. 8-13 with one PVC (the third beat from the end of the tracing). Comparison with Fig. 8-11 shows that the morphology of the PVC in Fig. 8-13 is identical to the QRS configuration for the tachydysrhythmia in Fig. 11. *Thus the patient must have been in ventricular tachycardia all along!*

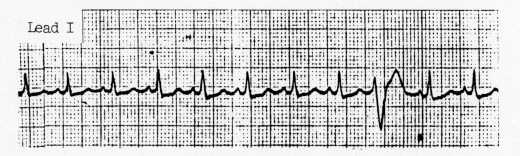

Fig. 8-13

Discussion

This case study brings out several important points. First, though ventricular tachycardia often rapidly degenerates into ventricular fibrillation, this is *not* always the case. This elderly woman was able to tolerate ventricular tachycardia for over an hour before spontaneously converting to sinus rhythm.

Second, although the QRS configuration of the tachydysrhythmia in Fig. 8-11 does not really appear bizarre, the QRS complex *is* wide and measures at least 0.12 second in duration. When confronted with a *regular, wide-complex tachydysrhythmia*, three diagnostic possibilities must be entertained.

• *SVT with preexisting bundle branch block*
• *SVT with aberrancy*
• *Ventricular tachycardia*

Ventricular tachycardia should always be assumed until proven otherwise. The error in this case was to assume a supraventricular etiology for the rhythm because of the almost normal-appearing QRS complex and the patient's stable hemodynamic state.

Scrutiny of the "rabbit-ear" configuration in lead V_1 of the 12-lead ECG (Fig. 8-12) offers an additional clue to the true mechanism of this dysrhythmia. With aberrancy the right rabbit ear is usually taller than the left. The fact that the left rabbit ear in lead V_1 is taller than the right suggests that the rhythm in Fig. 8-12 is ventricular tachycardia (see Table 5-1, p. 73).

Retrospectively, the patient should have been initially treated with *lidocaine*. If she were not to respond, *procainamide, bretylium,* or *synchronized cardioversion* at a low energy level (50 J) would have been appropriate.

The decision to opt for synchronized cardioversion in patients with ventricular tachycardia and the choice of energy level to employ depend on the urgency of the clinical situation. If a patient with ventricular tachycardia is hypotensive and unresponsive, cardioversion at a high energy level (200 J) should be undertaken without delay. On the other hand, in an alert patient who is hemodynamically stable, one or more boluses of lidocaine and/or the use of procainamide or bretylium may be tried before turning to cardioversion. If the patient acutely decompensates at any point during the administration of these antiarrhythmic agents, immediate cardioversion should be performed with 200 J.

CASE STUDY 4

A code blue is called in the hospital. You rush to the patient's room and find CPR in progress on an elderly woman. An IV line is in place, and monitoring leads are hooked up. As the ECG machine is turned on, the rhythm strip shown in Fig. 8-14 is recorded. All eyes turn toward you.

How do you interpret the rhythm? As the duly appointed director of the resuscitation effort, what would you do next?

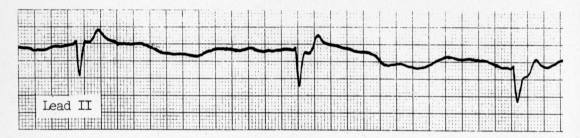

Fig. 8-14

ANALYSIS OF FIG. 8-14: No P waves are seen anywhere in the rhythm strip. The QRS complex appears somewhat widened, and the ventricular response is slow. With an R-R interval of 13 boxes, the ventricular rate is in the low 20s ($300 \div 13 = 23$ beats/min). This is a *slow idioventricular escape rhythm*.

1. Check for a pulse.
2. Have the nurse draw up 1 mg of *atropine*.
3. Try to obtain a capsule history of the patient's diagnosis and the events leading to the cardiopulmonary arrest.

Since only a slow and weak spontaneous pulse is palpable, you have your assistants resume CPR.

A nurse relates that the patient was admitted earlier that day for abdominal pain of 2-days' duration. The past medical history and review of systems are otherwise unremarkable, and the patient is on no medications. A 12-lead ECG was done on admission, but the official interpretation has not yet made its way into the chart.

The arrest itself was unwitnessed. The patient was found in an unresponsive state by a nurse on the floor, CPR was begun, and a code called.

One milligram of atropine has no effect on the rhythm shown in Fig. 8-14. What would you do at this point?

ANALYSIS
4. Administer an additional 1 mg of *atropine*.
5. Intubate the patient.
6. Consider giving the patient 1 ampule (50 mEq) of *sodium bicarbonate*.
7. Draw ABGs.
8. Obtain a complete blood count, serum electrolyte concentrations and a 12-lead ECG.

The standard dosing protocol for atropine sulfate calls for 0.5 mg to be given intravenously every 5 minutes to a maximum dose of 2 mg. This regimen would require 15 minutes for the full 2 mg of atropine to be given. With a slow ventricular escape rhythm and marked hemodynamic compromise, the drug can be safely administered in increments of 1 mg, thus significantly shortening the time for a therapeutic response. Additional dosing with atropine beyond the full amount of 2 mg is not felt to be beneficial.

Since the arrest in this patient was unwitnessed, the amount of time that the patient was unresponsive before resuscitation began is unknown. It was probably at least several minutes. In a hospital setting it would be reasonable to give 1 to 2 ampules of sodium bicarbonate initially, governing the further use of this drug by the results of ABGs.

Fig. 8-15 shows the patient's rhythm 1 minute after administration of the second dose of atropine. What has happened? Considering the patient is still unresponsive and has a palpable systolic blood pressure of only 60 mm Hg, how would you proceed?

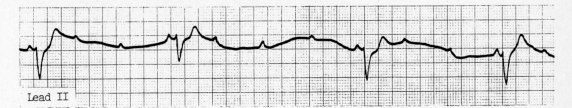

Lead II

Fig. 8-15

ANALYSIS OF FIG. 8-15: Although the QRS complex has not changed its configuration, the ventricular response is now somewhat irregular. Atrial activity has returned in the form of regularly occurring P waves at an atrial rate of about 90 beats/min (Fig. 8-16). Despite the irregularity of the ventricular response, *each QRS complex is preceded by a P wave with a fixed PR interval*. Because there is this definite relation between the QRS complex and its respective (immediately preceding) P wave, Fig. 8-16 cannot represent complete heart block. Since only one out of every three or four P waves is conducted, some type of advanced second-degree AV block is present. This is described as a *high-grade* or *high-degree AV block*.

Treatment of high-degree AV block is the same as treatment of Mobitz II second-degree AV block or third-degree AV block and involves atropine, isoproterenol, and pacemaker insertion.

9. Begin an *isoproterenol* infusion. Mix 1 mg in 250 ml of D_5W, and begin the infusion at 2 µg/min (30 drops/min). Titrate the rate of the drip upward as needed to increase heart rate and blood pressure.
10. Consult a cardiologist for emergency *pacemaker* insertion.

Traditionally, isoproterenol has been listed as the chronotropic agent of choice for the treatment of atropine-resistant bradydysrhythmias that are hemodynamically significant. However,

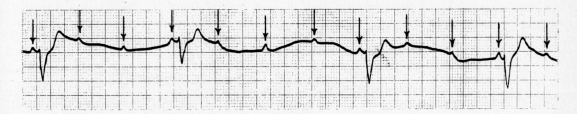

Fig. 8-16

the inotropic effect of isoproterenol results in a substantial increase in myocardial oxygen consumption that may potentiate ischemia and/or predispose the patient to ventricular dysrhythmias. In addition, the pure β-adrenergic stimulator effect of the drug lowers peripheral vascular resistance. This peripheral vasodilator action of isoproterenol sometimes overrides its inotropic effect and may result in hypotension with an overall decrease in cardiac output. At best isoproterenol should be used cautiously as a temporary stopgap measure to accelerate heart rate in hemodynamically significant bradydysrhythmias until definitive treatment (pacemaker insertion) can be accomplished.

Two other agents may be preferable to isoproterenol for treating bradydysrhythmias associated with hypotension. These drugs are *epinephrine* and *dopamine*. Both agents exert a potent inotropic effect that increases cardiac output, yet they increase blood pressure by augmenting peripheral vascular resistance.

When used to treat bradydysrhythmias, *epinephrine* may be administered as a continuous intravenous infusion. The infusion can be prepared in the same manner as for isoproterenol. Mix 1 mg of epinephrine in 250 ml of D_5W, and begin the infusion at 15 to 30 drops/min (1 to 2 $\mu g/min$). The speed of infusion may be titrated as needed to obtain the desired hemodynamic response.

The pharmacologic actions of *dopamine* are closely dose related. At low doses (1 to 2 $\mu g/kg/min$), the drug has a dopaminergic stimulator action that results in dilation of renal and mesenteric blood vessels. At doses of 2 to 10 $\mu g/kg/min$, the drug has a predominant β-receptor stimulator action that increases cardiac output. Between 10 and 20 $\mu g/kg/min$, the α-receptor stimulator action becomes more prominent and results in peripheral vasoconstriction. At doses above 20 $\mu g/kg/min$, the dopaminergic effect on the renal vasculature is reversed. The drug acts much like norepinephrine at this point.

An isoproterenol infusion is begun. Fig. 8-17 indicates the patient's response. What has happened?

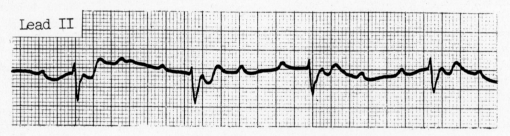

Fig. 8-17

ANALYSIS OF FIG. 8-17: Both the atrial rate and the ventricular response have increased when compared to Fig. 8-16. Each QRS complex is again preceded by a P wave, but from this small rhythm strip it is hard to be sure if the PR interval is constant. (In any case, the PR interval is different from what it was in Fig. 8-16.) This is either high-grade or complete AV block.

The isoproterenol infusion is continued, and a moment later the patient is observed to be in the rhythm shown in Fig. 8-18. Could this be ventricular tachycardia?

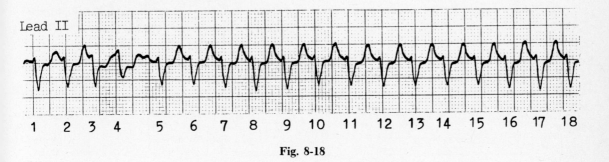

Lead II

1 2 3 4 5 6 7 8 9 10 11 12 13 14 15 16 17 18

Fig. 8-18

ANALYSIS OF FIG. 8-18: It is unlikely that the rhythm in Fig. 8-18 is ventricular tachycardia for two reasons.

- Although the QRS complex is wide, the configuration is identical to what it was in Fig. 8-16 in which conduction was supraventricular.
- A normal-appearing P wave precedes the onset of the tachydysrhythmia. (Because of the prematurity of beat 4 in Fig. 8-18, the T wave of this beat occurs earlier. This allows a distinct P wave to be identified in front of beat 5, whereas for the rest of the rhythm strip P waves are buried within the T waves.)

The rhythm in Fig. 8-18 thus is either *sinus tachycardia* or *PAT*. The ventricular response is 155 beats/min.

A nurse informs you that the patient's blood pressure has risen to 130/70 mm Hg with the rhythm in Fig. 8-18. What would you do next?

ANALYSIS

11. Turn down the isoproterenol infusion!

ABGs drawn just after the patient was intubated and given 1 ampule of sodium bicarbonate have returned and include the following:

$$PaCO_2 = 50 \text{ mm Hg}$$
$$PaO_2 = 70 \text{ mm Hg}$$
$$pH = 7.32$$
$$HCO_3^- = 25 \text{ mEq/L}$$

The admission ECG is finally brought to the floor. It suggests an anterior infarction of undetermined age. Comparison of this admission ECG with the 12-lead ECG that the technician has just recorded implies that the anterior infarction was acute and that this patient has now extended the area of injury.

By this time the cardiologist has taken over at the bedside and has already inserted a transvenous pacemaker. You are asked to remain by the ECG machine and monitor the patient's rhythm. However, the pulse is lost as you note the rhythm shown in Fig. 8-19. What has happened? What should you advise the cardiologist at the bedside?

ANALYSIS OF FIG. 8-19: Although regular pacemaker spikes are seen throughout the tracing at a rate of 100 beats/min, none of these spikes effectively capture the ventricles. As a result, the SVT continues for the first 10 beats of the rhythm strip and then stops abruptly after beat 10. Beat 11 is a sinus-conducted impulse with a different QRS configuration (the QRS is

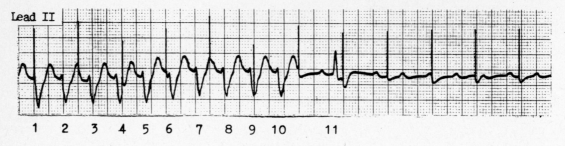

Fig. 8-19

narrow and upright compared to the left anterior hemiblock configuration that we have seen previously). This is followed by *ventricular standstill*. No QRS deflection follows the pacemaker spikes that occur after beat 11, reflecting the fact that cardiac pacing is *not* taking place.

12. Advise the cardiologist to manipulate the pacemaker wire until *capture* of the ventricles is effected.

The pacemaker is turned off while the pacing wire is advanced. Shortly after the pacemaker is turned back on, a strong femoral pulse is felt at

the bedside. Blood pressure is now 120/80 mm Hg. The rhythm is shown in Fig. 8-20. What do you see?

ANALYSIS OF FIG. 8-20: Ventricular standstill persists initially despite an atrial tachycardia of 160 beats/min. Midway through the strip, pacemaker spikes are seen at a rate of 120 beats/min. Effective ventricular capture is evidenced by the negative QRS deflection that follows these spikes. Since the patient's hemodynamic status has been stabilized, she can now be transferred to the coronary care unit.

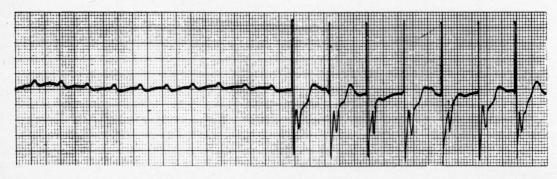

Fig. 8-20

Discussion

This case illustrates the difficulty encountered when one is called to the scene of a cardiac arrest on a patient who is not well known to the rescuer. In concert with initiation of the resuscitation attempt, high priority must be given to obtaining at least an abbreviated history of the patient. The elderly woman in this case study had been admitted earlier in the day for abdominal pain. Myocardial infarction was not initially suspected. It did not become apparent that she had in fact suffered an extensive anterior infarction until midway through the resuscitation procedure.

The diagnosis of acute myocardial infarction is usually suspected from a history of sudden, severe chest pain lasting at least 30 minutes, often with radiation to the neck or down the left arm. However, a significant number of patients do not relate a typical story, and up to 20% may have no chest pain at all! This is particularly true in the elderly who may experience stroke, a change in mental status, or as in this case an atypical location of pain. Retrospectively, had the diagnosis of infarction been entertained on admission, this patient's ECG would have been reviewed earlier, and she would have been admitted to an intensive care unit at the outset.

Assuming that the woman in this case study was active and functional before her admission, the aggressive approach to resuscitation that was pursued was appropriate. A different scenario might be imagined in which one walks into the code of an elderly bedridden patient with terminal metastatic disease for whom specific orders not to resuscitate are indicated on the chart. An unfortunate outcome might result if the hospital staff involved in the resuscitation were not aware of these orders and/or made no attempt to seek out such information about the patient. The code director must assume responsibility for securing whatever historical information is needed to effectively manage the code.

The ABGs in this case study were drawn shortly after intubation. The results were reported as follows:

$Pa_{CO_2} = 50$ mm Hg

$Pa_{O_2} = 70$ mm Hg

$pH = 7.32$

$HCO_3^- = 25$ mEq/L

How did you interpret these results?

ANALYSIS: There is *hypoxemia* and a pure *respiratory acidosis. (An acute change in Pa_{CO_2} of 10 mm Hg is associated with an approximate change in pH of 0.08 in the opposite direction.* Since the Pa_{CO_2} has increased from 40 to 50 mm Hg in this patient, one would expect her pH to decrease by 0.08 units to 7.32 if these results could be solely attributed to the hypoventilation that existed before intubation.) There is *no* metabolic component to the acidosis, since the HCO_3^- is normal (25 mEq/L). (The metabolic component that did exist must have been corrected by the ampule of sodium bicarbonate that was administered.)

It is interesting that this patient only required 1 ampule of sodium bicarbonate. In the past much higher doses were used, which led to a disturbing incidence of iatrogenic alkalosis. A key factor in avoiding such overdosing is to remember when in the sequence of events ABGs are drawn. In this case study the patient had been intubated just before ABGs were obtained. Simply increasing ventilation would be expected to correct the hypercapnia and normalize the pH. No additional sodium bicarbonate should be needed.

CASE STUDY 5

A 65-year-old man comes to the emergency department for chest pain. You are taking a history from him as an IV line is established and monitoring leads are applied. The patient suddenly loses consciousness and becomes pulseless. You look up at the monitor and see the rhythm shown in Fig. 8-21. What do you do?

ANALYSIS OF FIG. 8-21: A regular, wide complex tachydysrhythmia is present at a rate of about 170 beats/min. *Ventricular tachycardia* must be assumed until proven otherwise. Since the patient is pulseless, the treatment is the same as for ventricular fibrillation.

1. Deliver a *precordial thump.*
2. Apply *countershock* with *200 J* of delivered energy.

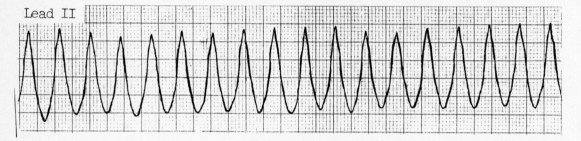

Fig. 8-21

The only indication for the precordial thump in cardiopulmonary arrest is at the onset of monitored ventricular tachycardia or ventricular fibrillation. This situation exists in this case.

If the patient does not respond to the precordial thump, countershock rather than synchronized cardioversion would be preferred for pulseless ventricular tachycardia.

Following countershock the rhythm shown in Fig. 8-22 appears on the monitor. What is this rhythm? How would you proceed?

ANALYSIS OF FIG. 8-22: Once again the QRS complex is wide. However, as opposed to Fig. 8-21, the rhythm is irregularly irregular. This suggests that the rhythm in Fig. 8-22 is not ventricular tachycardia but instead might represent *atrial fibrillation* with *preexisting bundle branch block.*

3. Check for a pulse and blood pressure.

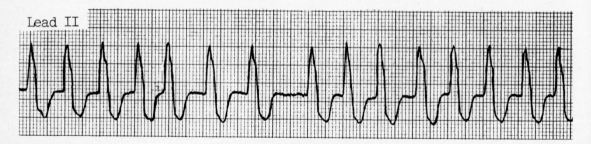

Fig. 8-22

The patient has a strong pulse and a systolic blood pressure of 110 mm Hg, but before you can take a deep breath, the monitor changes to the rhythm shown in Fig. 8-23. The pulse is lost. What do you do?

ANALYSIS OF FIG. 8-23: The patient is now in *ventricular fibrillation*.

4. Apply countershock with 200 J.

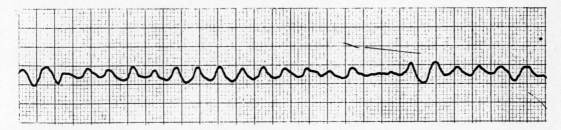

Fig. 8-23

Following countershock, Fig. 8-24 is recorded. What do you do next?

ANALYSIS OF FIG. 8-24: A series of irregular and seemingly narrow complexes is seen in Fig. 8-24. In areas these complexes occur at a rate that exceeds 300 beats/min! No real rhythm has a ventricular response this fast. Thus Fig. 8-24 must be *artifactual*.

5. Look for the source of artifact, and obtain another rhythm strip.

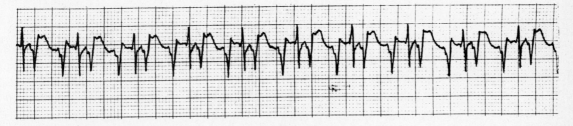

Fig. 8-24

A loose monitoring lead is secured, and the rhythm in Fig. 8-25 is now seen on the monitor. A strong femoral pulse returns, but the patient is still unresponsive. What is the rhythm?

ANALYSIS OF FIG. 8-25: The QRS complex has narrowed, and the rhythm is irregularly irregular. This is *atrial fibrillation* with a *rapid ventricular response*.

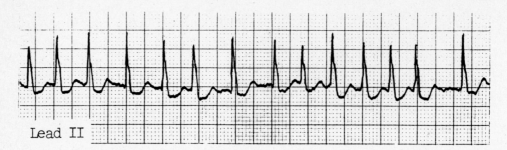

Lead II

Fig. 8-25

A blood pressure of 100/70 mm Hg is obtained, and the patient begins breathing on his own. Fig. 8-26 signals the appearance of two types of abnormal looking complexes (i.e., beats 3, 4, 22, and 6 to 9). How do you interpret this rhythm strip? Is any treatment indicated?

ANALYSIS OF FIG. 8-26: The underlying rhythm is irregularly irregular, and no P waves are evident. This is again *atrial fibrillation* with a *rapid ventricular response*. Since Fig. 8-26 is taken from lead II rather than a right-sided monitoring lead, analyzing the QRS morphology of the anomalous beats is not helpful in distinguishing PVCs from aberrantly conducted beats. However, the QRS complexes of beats 6 to 9 are not really wide, and they

have a similar initial deflection to the normally conducted beats. These beats also maintain the cadence of the atrial fibrillation (the R-R interval varies, and the run ends as abruptly as it begins), suggesting that they are *aberrantly conducted*.

In contrast, beats 3, 4, and 22 are wider and begin with an initial negative deflection that is opposite to that of the normally conducted beats. A postectopic pause follows beat 22. Beats 3, 4, and 22 are *PVCs*.

6. Give the patient a 75 mg bolus of *lidocaine*, and begin an infusion at 2 mg/min.
7. Consider the use of *digoxin* in an attempt to slow the ventricular response.

or

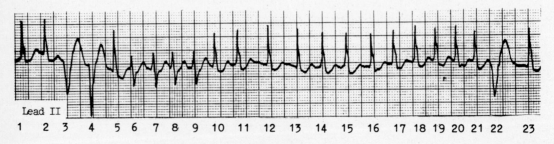

Lead II

1 2 3 4 5 6 7 8 9 10 11 12 13 14 15 16 17 18 19 20 21 22 23

Fig. 8-26

8. Use *cardioversion* on the patient.

Even without the PVCs seen in Fig. 8-26, lidocaine would be indicated as a prophylactic measure to prevent the recurrence of ventricular tachycardia or ventricular fibrillation.

Digoxin is not recommended for treatment of congestive heart failure with acute myocardial infarction. The risk of developing toxicity is greater in this setting, and other agents (diuretics, morphine sulfate, vasodilators) are usually more effective in the initial treatment. However, digoxin remains an excellent agent for slowing the ventricular response to atrial flutter or fibrillation regardless of the setting in which these atrial tachydysrhythmias occur.

In the nondigitalized patient, an initial loading dose of 0.25 to 0.50 mg is administered intravenously. This should be followed every 2 to 6 hours with additional 0.125 to 0.250 mg IV increments until a total loading dose of 0.75 to 1.50 mg has been administered. This loading schedule can be adjusted according to the ventricular response, although more cautious dosing is advised with acute ischemia.

Although *synchronized cardioversion* is the treatment of choice for hemodynamically significant atrial tachydysrhythmias, the stable blood pressure of the patient in this case study makes digitalization a reasonable choice over cardioversion. (However, if the patient's hemodynamic status were to subsequently deteriorate, the emergency care provider should realize that cardioversion carries an increased risk in patients receiving digitalis.)

Finally, intravenous *verapamil* may be used as an alternative agent to digoxin for slowing the ventricular response of atrial fibrillation or flutter. Five to ten milligrams (0.075 to 0.150 mg/kg) are administered intravenously over a 1- to 2-minute period (or even slower in the elderly). This dose may be repeated in 30 minutes. Unlike PSVT, for which verapamil successfully restores sinus rhythm in the overwhelming majority of cases, the drug only occasionally converts atrial fibrillation or flutter to sinus rhythm. The ventricular response is slowed, but the effect is usually only transient.

The patient is given an initial IV bolus of 0.25 mg of digoxin. A 12-lead ECG reveals an acute inferior injury current, and he is transferred to the coronary care unit. Two hours later another 0.25 mg of digoxin is given. The patient is now awake, alert, without chest pain, and hemodynamically stable. His rhythm is shown in Fig. 8-27. What is your interpretation?

ANALYSIS OF FIG. 8-27: The rhythm is still atrial fibrillation but with a slower ventricular response. The ventricular ectopy has disappeared.

The patient is maintained on a lidocaine infusion for 24 hours and receives an additional 0.25 mg of digoxin over this period. An inferior infarction evolves, but the patient continues to do well and is discharged from the coronary care unit 2 days later on a maintenance dosage of 0.25 mg of digoxin daily.

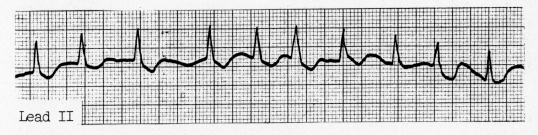

Lead II

Fig. 8-27

CASE STUDY 6

A cardiopulmonary arrest is called on a 60-year-old woman in the intensive care unit. You arrive to find CPR in progress and the patient already intubated. The patient looks like she weighs about 170 pounds. A number of nurses and physicians are furiously working around the bedside, but no one has assumed direction of the code. You decide to station yourself by the ECG machine and observe the rhythm shown in Fig. 8-28. How would you advise the bedside team?

ANALYSIS OF FIG. 8-28: The ventricular response is slow and regular at about 30 beats/min, but no P waves are seen. The QRS complex is narrow, suggesting the *escape* focus as originating from low down in the conduction system. What might you want to know about the patient and/or the events that have transpired so far?

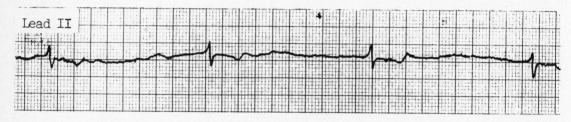

Fig. 8-28

1. Is there a pulse? What is the blood pressure?
2. Does anyone know about the patient's history or the events leading up to the code?
3. Was the arrest witnessed? Have any drugs been given?

A slow, weak pulse is felt at the bedside, and a systolic blood pressure of 60 mm Hg is obtained by palpation. The patient had been admitted a day earlier for deep venous thrombophlebitis. The arrest was witnessed, and CPR was begun promptly. *Endotracheal intubation* was accomplished within the first minute of the arrest, and 1 mg of *atropine* has already been given.

The respiratory therapist hands you the first set of ABGs that were drawn about a minute after the patient was intubated. The following are the readings:

$$pH = 7.13$$
$$Pa_{O_2} = 45 \text{ mm Hg}$$
$$Pa_{CO_2} = 55 \text{ mm Hg}$$
$$HCO_3^- = 16 \text{ mEq/L}$$

How would you interpret these results? What should be done next?

ANALYSIS: The ABGs reflect a combined *metabolic* and *respiratory acidosis* with significant *hypoxemia*. However, both the Pa_{O_2} and pH values are much lower than one would expect for a patient in whom CPR and endotracheal intubation were promptly carried out.

4. Listen for breath sounds.
5. Administer 1 to 2 ampules of *sodium bicarbonate*.
6. Consider the possibility of pulmonary embolism as an etiology for the marked hypoxemia in view of the admitting diagnosis.

Breath sounds are greatly diminished on the left side. They normalize after the endotracheal tube is withdrawn slightly. The patient's pulse picks up as you observe the rhythm shown in Fig. 8-29. Blood pressure is now 100/70 mm Hg. What is the rhythm, and what would you do?

ANALYSIS OF FIG. 8-29: The patient is now in a *junctional rhythm* at 65 beats/min.

7. Catch your breath. No treatment is needed for a patient in junctional rhythm who is hemodynamically stable.
8. Repeat the ABGs now that the endotracheal tube is repositioned.

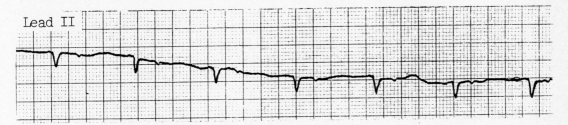

Fig. 8-29

Moments later you observe in succession the rhythms shown in Figs. 8-30 and 8-31. The patient's blood pressure remains 100/70 mm Hg. What has happened? What should be done?

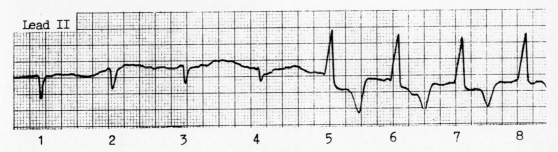

Fig. 8-30

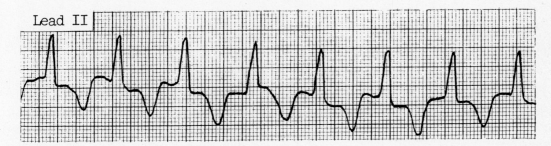

Fig. 8-31

ANALYSIS OF FIGS. 8-30 AND 8-31: No P waves are seen in either strip. The junctional rhythm seen earlier in Fig. 8-29 continues for the first four beats in Fig. 8-30. Beat 5 occurs early and initiates a regular rhythm with a wider QRS complex of a different configuration. This is an accelerated idioventricular rhythm (AIVR); it speeds up slightly but continues throughout Fig. 8-31.

9. Do nothing. *Benign neglect* is the treatment of choice.

AIVR is commonly observed with acute myocardial infarction or cardiopulmonary arrest. It is defined as the occurrence of three or more consecutive QRS complexes of ventricular origin with a rate between 50 and 100 beats/min. Also known as "slow ventricular tachycardia," AIVR does not usually result in the adverse hemodynamic effects of the more rapid ventricular tachydysrhythmias. When confronted with this rhythm, one may choose among the following three therapeutic options:
• *Cautious observation*
• *Suppression of the rhythm with lidocaine or countershock*
• *Acceleration of the supraventricular pacemaker with atropine*

AIVR may occur when the ventricular rate overrides the supraventricular pacemaker. This is the case in Fig. 8-30 in which a junctional rhythm at 65 beats/min is superceded by AIVR at 70 beats/min. If the patient remains asymptomatic and hemodynamically stable, *no treatment* is needed. If hypotension occurs, the preferred therapy is to give *atropine* in an attempt to stimulate the supraventricular pacemaker to overtake the ventricular rhythm.

It is important to emphasize that AIVR may arise as an escape rhythm for a failing SA or AV node. Under these circumstances, suppression of the ventricular escape rhythm with *lidocaine* may result in ventricular standstill if no supraventricular pacemaker is able to take over. It is for this reason that treatment of AIVR with lidocaine is generally *not* recommended. Similarly, one would not want to use countershock with this rhythm in a patient who is hemodynamically stable.

The patient's blood pressure drops to a palpable systolic reading of 70 mm Hg with the rhythm shown in Fig. 8-31. CPR is restarted, and she is given 1 mg of *atropine*. (A total of 2 mg of atropine has now been given.) Fig. 8-32 shows her response. What has happened?

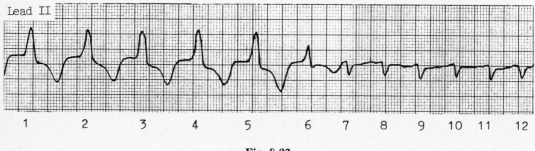

Fig. 8-32

ANALYSIS OF FIG. 8-32: AIVR continues for the first five beats in Fig. 8-32 until an accelerated supraventricular pacemaker takes over at a rate of 130 beats/min (beats 7 to 12). This is most likely *junctional tachycardia*, since no P waves are evident and the QRS configuration is similar to that of the junctional rhythm in Fig. 8-29. Beat 6 demonstrates a QRS configuration that is intermediate between the accelerated idioventricular beats and the junctional beats. This complex is a *fusion beat*.

A moment later the rhythm shown in Fig. 8-33 is observed. This is associated with only a weak pulse without an obtainable blood pressure. How would you proceed?

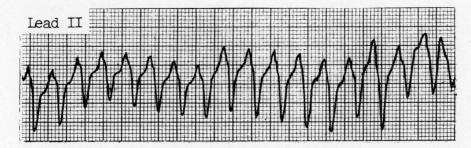

Fig. 8-33

ANALYSIS OF FIG. 8-33: A regular tachydysrhythmia at a rate of 220 beats/min is seen in Fig. 8-33. Although the QRS configuration is somewhat similar to that of the junctional tachycardia seen in beats 7 to 12 of Fig. 8-32, the QRS complex is wider and deeper, raising the possibility that this may be ventricular tachycardia. Failure to identify P waves does not assist in resolving this dilemma. *One cannot absolutely differentiate between PJT with aberrant conduction and ventricular tachycardia from inspection of Fig. 8-33.* However, in the clinical context of hemodynamic compromise, treatment of this tachydysrhythmia does *not* depend on this differentiation. Immediate *synchronized cardioversion* is advised regardless of whether a supraventricular or ventricular etiology exists.

10. Use *cardioversion* with 100 to 200 J of delivered energy.

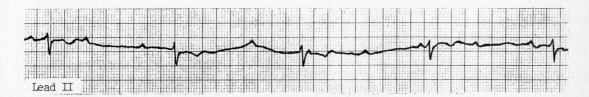

Fig. 8-34

Cardioversion results in the rhythm shown in Fig. 8-34. This is associated with a weak pulse and a systolic blood pressure of 60 mm Hg. What is the rhythm? What treatment would you recommend?

ANALYSIS OF FIG. 8-34: The QRS complex is narrow, and the ventricular response is regular at 32 beats/min. The atrial rate is also regular at 70 beats/min (arrows in Fig. 8-35), but P waves are totally unrelated to the QRS complex (the PR interval constantly changes). This is *complete AV block*. (The reason a P wave is not evident immediately following the QRS complex of beat 2 in Fig. 8-35 is that it is contained within the ST segment of this beat. The dotted arrow indicates where this P wave would be expected to occur.)

11. Consult a cardiologist for emergency *pacemaker insertion.*
12. Start an infusion with either *isoproterenol, dopamine,* or *epinephrine.*

Definitive treatment for complete AV block is cardiac pacing. Until a physician capable of inserting a pacemaker arrives, however, an attempt must be made to restore adequate perfusion. Since administration of the full dose of atropine (2 mg) has not been successful, attention should be directed to starting an IV infusion with one of the three agents listed in instruction 12.

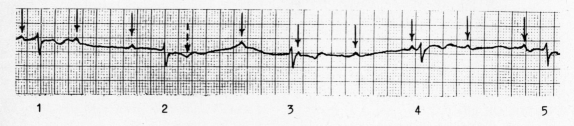

Fig. 8-35

You receive the message that the cardiologist will be there in about 10 minutes. Meanwhile an isoproterenol drip is started at an initial infusion rate of 2μg/min. As the infusion rate is titrated upward, the pulse is suddenly lost, and the rhythm shown in Fig. 8-36 supervenes. What is the diagnosis? What would be the recommended treatment?

ANALYSIS OF FIG. 8-36: The rhythm is *ventricular fibrillation.*

13. Apply countershock with 200 J.

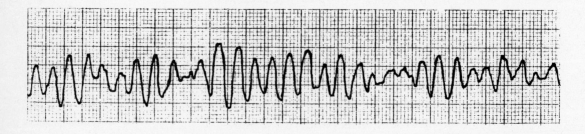

Fig. 8-36

Countershock results in the rhythm shown in Fig. 8-37. What would be the treatment?

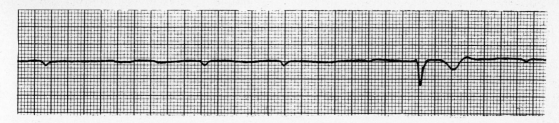

Fig. 8-37

ANALYSIS OF FIG. 8-37: With the exception of an isolated QRS complex, this is *ventricular standstill*. Treatment is the same as for asystole.

14. Resume CPR.
15. Administer 1 mg of *epinephrine* IV.
16. Consider additional sodium bicarbonate.

The repeat ABGs drawn after repositioning the endotracheal tube are returned with the following readings:

$$pH = 7.31$$
$$PaO_2 = 120 \text{ mm Hg}$$
$$PaCO_2 = 37 \text{ mm Hg}$$
$$HCO_3^- = 19 \text{ mEq/L}$$

Considering these results, do you feel that the use of sodium bicarbonate is indicated?

ANALYSIS: The hypoxemia present in the first set of ABGs has been corrected, and only a mild metabolic acidosis remains. Additional bicarbonate is probably *not* warranted at this point.

What other therapeutic alternatives should be considered if the rhythm shown in Fig. 8-37 does not respond to 1 mg of epinephrine?

ANALYSIS
17. Administer atropine.
18. Administer calcium chloride.
19. Restart the isoproterenol infusion if 1 mg of epinephrine is ineffective.
20. Administer additional *epinephrine*.
21. Consider pacemaker insertion. (The cardiologist is still 5 minutes away.)

Atropine may occasionally be effective in asystole because of the fact that there is some parasympathetic innervation of the ventricles. One would not expect additional atropine to be of benefit in this case, since the full dose of atropine has already been given.

Calcium chloride has been recommended in the past for EMD and asystole, yet recent studies suggest that ultimate patient survival is not improved and may actually be adversely affected by the use of this drug. As a result, one might reserve calcium chloride until other agents have been tried and have failed.

Isoproterenol is a potent chronotropic and inotropic agent, but it should probably not be used during cardiovascular collapse (asystole, EMD, ventricular fibrillation) because of its potentially detrimental effect on coronary blood flow. Coronary artery blood flow occurs principally during diastole. Beta-adrenergic stimulating agents like isoproterenol produce peripheral vasodilation that lowers diastolic blood pressure and impairs coronary flow. Alpha-adrenergic stimulating agents such as *epinephrine* increase systemic vascular resistance and favor coronary flow. If the rhythm shown in Fig. 8-37 does not respond to 1 ampule of epinephrine, administration of a second (and third) ampule would probably be the treatment of choice.

Two ampules (2 mg) of epinephrine given over the next few minutes produce the ventricular response shown in Fig. 8-38. How would you interpret this rhythm?

ANALYSIS OF FIG. 8-38: Beats 1 and 2 represent a slow idioventricular response at a rate of 20 beats/min. Beats 3 to 5 demonstrate progressive narrowing of the QRS complex and acceleration of the heart rate as the location of the escape focus changes.

Fig. 8-38 evolves into the rhythm shown in Fig. 8-39. Blood pressure is 70/40 mm Hg. What would you do at this point?

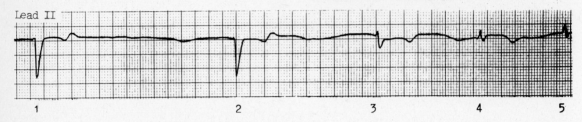

Fig. 8-38

ANALYSIS OF FIG. 8-39: Sinus rhythm at a rate of 60 beats/min is present in Fig. 8-39.

22. Begin an *epinephrine infusion*. Mix 1 ampule (1 mg) in 250 ml of D_5W, and begin the drip at 15 to 30 drops/min (1 to 2 μg/min).

or

23. Begin a *dopamine infusion*. Mix 1 ampule (200 mg) in 250 ml of D_5W, and begin the drip at 15 to 30 drops/min (about 2 to 5 μg/kg/min).

Increase the infusion rate of the drug chosen as needed, according to the blood pressure response.

and

24. Administer a 75 mg bolus of *lidocaine*, and begin an infusion at 2 mg/min.

Since *epinephrine* was effective in obtaining a rhythm with a pulse, it would be reasonable to choose this drug for a maintenance infusion. Otherwise, *dopamine* is probably the therapeutic agent of choice for treating cardiogenic shock. At infusion rates between 2 to 10 μg/kg/min, this drug primarily acts as an inotropic agent without the marked chronotropic effect of isoproterenol. At doses above 20 μg/kg/min, it acts much like norepinephrine.

The use of *lidocaine* is indicated as a prophylactic measure to prevent the recurrence of ventricular fibrillation. One might want to wait until the blood pressure responds to the pressor chosen before initiating the lidocaine infusion.

The patient's blood pressure increases to 110/80 mm Hg on dopamine, and she begins to breathe on her own.

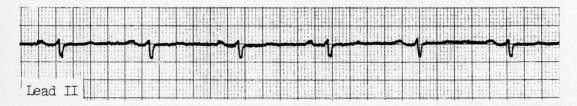

Fig. 8-39

CASE STUDY 7

A previously healthy 45-year-old man comes to the emergency department complaining of severe crushing chest pain that has lasted 1 hour. He is diaphoretic and has a blood pressure of 90/60 mm Hg. A 12-lead ECG demonstrates an acute inferior injury current, and his rhythm is shown in Fig. 8-40. How would you interpret this rhythm strip?

ANALYSIS OF FIG. 8-40: The ventricular response in Fig. 8-40 is regular at a rate of 53 beats/min, and each QRS complex is preceded by a P wave with a fixed PR interval of 0.26 second. The terminal portion of each T wave appears notched, raising the question of whether or not an additional nonconducted P wave may be present.

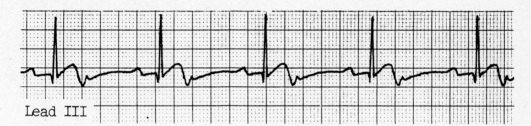

Lead III

Fig. 8-40

A helpful technique for determining if 2:1 AV conduction exists is to set one's calipers at one half the R-R interval (0.58 second in Fig. 8-41) and then see if P waves march out at this setting. When this is done and calipers are walked out, the notch in the terminal portion of the T wave is seen to occur precisely on time. Thus the atrial rate in Fig. 8-40 is 106 beats/min and *second-degree AV block* with *2:1 AV conduction* is present (every other P wave is not conducted). Is the second-degree AV block of the Mobitz I or Mobitz II variety?

ANALYSIS: Although the PR interval preceding each QRS complex is fixed, suggesting Mobitz II second-degree AV block, *one cannot rule out Mobitz I in the presence of 2:1 AV conduction.* Since only one QRS complex is conducted before a beat is dropped, the opportunity for the PR interval to progressively lengthen before dropping a beat never exists.

The following three features suggest that the rhythm in Fig. 8-40 is more likely to be *Mobitz I* than Mobitz II:

• The QRS complex is narrow.

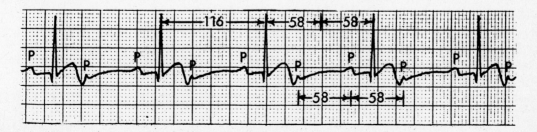

Fig. 8-41

- First-degree AV block is present.
- The ECG suggests acute inferior infarction.

Whereas the site of the conduction disturbance in Mobitz I is at the AV node, the block in *Mobitz II* occurs lower down in the conduction system. As a result, the QRS complex is usually of normal duration in Mobitz I and widened with Mobitz II. The PR interval is frequently normal with Mobitz II but is often prolonged with Mobitz I. Statistically with acute inferior infarction, Mobitz I is much more common than is Mobitz II. (See Table 7-1 on p. 96.)

Distinguishing between Mobitz II and Mobitz I second-degree AV block is important, since pacemaker insertion is essential for the former but is rarely required for the latter. Although the previously noted features are not hard and fast rules for making this differentia-

tion, they are helpful guidelines to use when confronted with a second-degree AV block that manifests 2:1 AV conduction.

The patient is given supplemental *oxygen* by nasal cannula, and an IV line is established. His pain is virtually relieved by 5 mg of IV *morphine sulfate*, and he is resting comfortably as the rhythm shown in Fig. 8-42 is recorded on the monitor. Blood pressure is 95/60 mm Hg. Has the patient gone into complete AV block?

ANALYSIS OF FIG. 8-42: Regularly occurring P waves (at an atrial rate of 85 beats/min) are seen to march through this rhythm strip without apparent relation to the QRS complex. Yet the R-R interval is *not* regular. This makes it unlikely that complete AV block is present, since third-degree AV block is most often associated with regularity of the ventricular response.

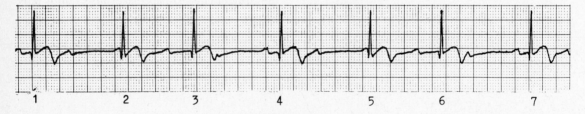

Fig. 8-42

Fig. 8-43 demonstrates the regularity of the atrial rate in this rhythm. The PR interval preceding beats 2 and 5 is definitely too short to conduct (arrows in Fig. 8-43). Beats 2 and 5

must therefore be *junctional beats*. Since the R-R interval preceding these beats is about the same as the R-R interval between beats 3 and 4 and 6 and 7, it is likely that this constant R-R interval reflects a junctional escape

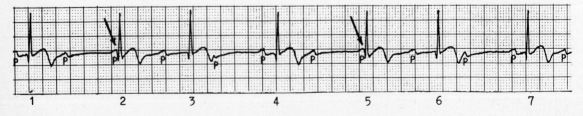

Fig. 8-43

rhythm at 47 beats/min. The reason the R-R interval shortens for beats 3 and 6 is that these beats are sinus conducted, albeit with first-degree AV block. Thus *intermittent AV dissociation* is present rather than complete AV block. Although this mechanism is rather complex, the important point to realize is that the rhythm in Fig. 8-42 is *not* complete AV block and does *not* necessarily require a pace-maker (provided that the ventricular response of the junctional escape focus is adequate to maintain a stable blood pressure).

A moment later the rhythm shown in Fig. 8-44 is observed on the monitor. The patient remains comfortable. Blood pressure is 100/70 mm Hg. What is the rhythm? Is treatment indicated?

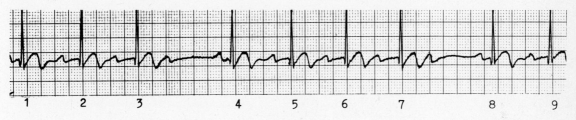

Fig. 8-44

ANALYSIS OF FIG. 8-44: Two beats are dropped in Fig. 8-44 (the P waves following beats 3 and 7 are not conducted). The atrial rate is regular at 80 beats/min (Fig. 8-45), and each QRS complex is preceded by a P wave with a progressively longer PR interval until a P wave is blocked. This is *second-degree AV block, Mobitz I (Wenckebach)*. No treatment is indicated, since the patient is hemodynamically stable.

With acute inferior infarction, the occurrence of Mobitz I AV block is usually the result of ischemia of the AV node. The block is most often transient, and no treatment is needed if the patient is asymptomatic and hemodynamically stable. If hypotension supervenes, atropine is the drug of choice. Pacemaker insertion is only necessary for those uncommon cases of Wenckebach in which hypotension persists despite vagolytic doses of atropine and correction of any existing intravascular volume deficit.

Even third-degree AV block may occur with inferior myocardial infarction as the result of ischemia of the AV node. If a junctional escape rhythm takes over at an adequate ventricular response to maintain hemodynamic stability, one may elect to withhold pacemaker insertion and carefully observe the patient even though there is complete AV block. This differs significantly from the management of inferior infarc-

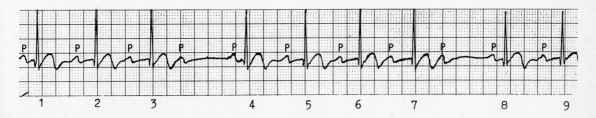

Fig. 8-45

tion with third-degree AV block and a slow idioventricular escape rhythm or third-degree AV block of any kind that occurs with anterior infarction. In both of these latter situations, insertion of a prophylactic pacemaker is mandatory. (See Table 7-2 on p. 101.)

This patient was given *prophylactic lidocaine* initially and was transferred to the coronary care unit. He reverted to sinus rhythm several hours later and suffered no further complications for the remainder of his hospital stay.

Discussion

The fact that Wenckebach is clearly present in Fig. 8-44 is further evidence supporting the assumption that the second-degree AV block seen earlier in Fig. 8-40 is also Mobitz I. It is extremely unusual for a patient to switch back and forth from Mobitz II to Mobitz I.

It is interesting that the atrial rate progressively decreases from Figs. 8-40 to 8-44. Whereas at an atrial rate of 106 beats/min (Fig. 8-40) only 2:1 AV conduction is possible, much better AV conduction occurs when the atrial rate slows down (Fig. 8-44).

Lidocaine is indicated as a prophylactic measure in this patient despite the absence of any ectopic activity because of the following:

- The index of suspicion for acute infarction is extremely high.
- The patient is seen within the first few hours of the onset of his symptoms.
- The patient is well under 70 years old. The risk of lidocaine toxicity is greater in older patients, whereas the incidence of primary ventricular fibrillation is much less.

Caution in the administration of lidocaine is advised in this patient because of the Mobitz I second-degree AV conduction disorder.

CASE STUDY 8

A 70-year-old woman collapses at home. The arrest is witnessed by her son who initiates CPR and activates the EMS. You are among the ambulance crew dispatched to the patient's home. On your arrival the patient is unresponsive, and the son is still doing one-rescuer CPR. Quick-look paddles applied to the patient's chest reveal the rhythm shown in Fig. 8-46. How would you proceed?

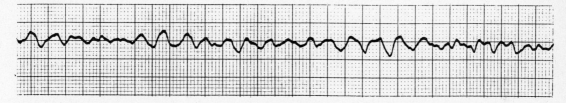

Fig. 8-46

ANALYSIS OF FIG. 8-46: The patient is in ventricular fibrillation.

1. Defibrillate with *200 J* of delivered energy.

Fig. 8-47 reveals the patient's response to initial defibrillation. What to you do next?

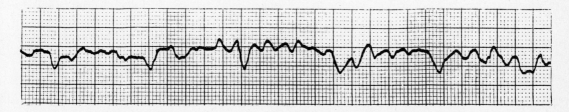

Fig. 8-47

ANALYSIS OF FIG. 8-47: The patient is still in ventricular fibrillation.

2. Immediately *defibrillate again* with *200 J*.

A weak pulse is now felt, and the rhythm shown in Fig. 8-48 is observed. What is the diagnosis? What is the recommended treatment?

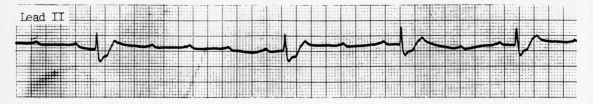

Fig. 8-48

ANALYSIS OF FIG. 8-48: Regular P waves are seen to march through the rhythm strip with an atrial rate of 115 beats/min. The QRS is wide and the ventricular rate slow and irregular, yet each QRS complex is preceded by a P wave with a fixed PR interval. Since a constant relation is maintained between each QRS complex and its preceding P wave, the rhythm is *not* complete AV block but rather an *advanced form* of *second-degree AV block*.

3. Resume CPR.
4. Intubate the patient.
5. Establish IV access.
6. Hook up monitoring leads to the patient.

The patient is easily intubated but *no one is able to secure an IV line*. The rhythm shown in Fig. 8-48 persists. What would you do at this point?

ANALYSIS
7. Administer 1 mg of *atropine* (the contents of one 10 ml prefilled syringe) *intratracheally*, and follow this with several forceful insufflations to drive the drug distally into the respiratory tree where absorption may take place.

and/or

8. Administer 1 mg of *epinephrine* (one 10 ml syringe of a 1:10,000 solution) *intratracheally*, followed by several forceful insufflations.

Recent attention has focused on the intratracheal administration of drugs during cardiopulmonary arrest when IV access cannot be established. Absorption across bronchoalveolar structures has been shown to be excellent for a number of medications including *atropine*, *lidocaine*, and *epinephrine*. (Use of the mnemonic *ALE* may help recall these drugs.) It is important to dilute the agent to a volume of at least 5 to 10 ml and to follow instillation of the intratracheal bolus by several forceful insufflations to assure adequate distribution of drug to the distal respiratory tree. When administered in this manner, intratracheal medications are rapidly absorbed into the bloodstream and exert a sustained effect that may exceed the duration of the action of drugs injected intravenously. (Unfortunately, sodium bicarbonate *cannot* be given by the intratracheal route.)

Instillation of a 1 mg intratracheal bolus of *atropine* results in the rhythm shown in Fig. 8-49. What has happened?

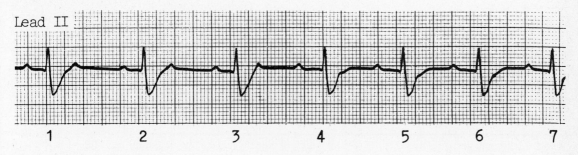

Fig. 8-49

ANALYSIS OF FIG. 8-49: The R-R interval progressively decreases in Fig. 8-49 as the ventricular response increases. Compared to Fig. 8-48, AV conduction has improved so that every other P wave is now conducted. Note how the nonconducted P wave notches the terminal portion of the T wave for beats 1 to 3. With progressive acceleration of the atrial rate, the nonconducted P wave becomes buried within the ST segment of beats 4 to 7 (broken arrows in Fig. 8-50).

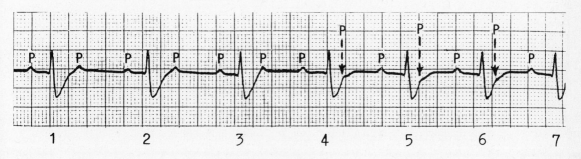

Fig. 8-50

A moment later the rhythm shown in Fig. 8-51 is observed on the monitor. How should you proceed? (No one has yet been able to secure an IV line.)

ANALYSIS OF FIG. 8-51: The first five beats in Fig. 8-51 demonstrate an SVT that degenerates into ventricular fibrillation.

9. Administer a *precordial thump*.

and/or

10. *Defibrillate* with 200 to 360 J.

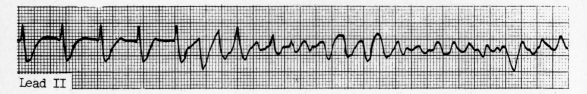

Lead II

Fig. 8-51

Since 200 J effectively converted the patient out of ventricular fibrillation earlier, it would be reasonable to use the same energy level again. Alternatively, one might choose to defibrillate the patient with the maximum delivered energy (360 J).

Fig. 8-52 illustrates the response to defibrillation. A palpable pulse and a systolic blood pressure of 80 mm Hg is associated with this rhythm. How would you interpret the tracing?

ANALYSIS OF FIG. 8-52: Tachydysrhythmias with two different QRS morphologies are evident in this rhythm strip. The initial tachycardia (beats 1 to 6 and 8 to 10) is most likely supraventricular. Although the QRS complex is wide, its configuration is identical to that shown earlier in Figs. 8-48 and 8-49 where the constant PR interval confirmed supraventricular conduction. Since no P waves can be identified, one cannot differentiate between sinus tachycardia (with P waves hidden within the ST segment), PAT, and PJT. The rate is 140 beats/min.

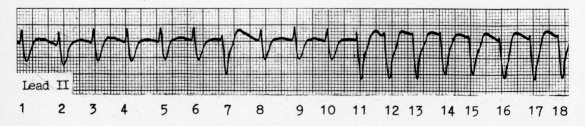

Lead II

1 2 3 4 5 6 7 8 9 10 11 12 13 14 15 16 17 18

Fig. 8-52

Beat 7 is probably a PVC. It is wide, premature, and the R-R interval enclosing it constitutes a full compensatory pause. Since the tachydysrhythmia beginning with beat 11 demonstrates a QRS configuration identical to that of this PVC, ventricular tachycardia at a rate of 160 beats/min should be assumed for beats 11 to 18.

An IV line is finally started. Considering that a systolic blood pressure of 80 mm Hg has been maintained during the run of ventricular tachycardia, what therapeutic options might you exercise? (The patient weighs about 50 kg.)

ANALYSIS

11. Administer a 50 to 75 mg IV bolus of *lidocaine*, and begin an infusion at a rate of 2 mg/min.

or

12. Mix 1 ampule (500 mg) of *bretylium* in 50 ml of D_5W, and infuse over a 10-minute period.

or

13. Use *cardioversion* on the patient with *200 J*.

The patient is given a 75 mg bolus of *lidocaine*, and an infusion is begun. Despite this, the pulse is lost, and the rhythm shown in Fig. 8-53 is observed. What would you do now?

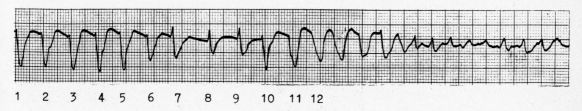

1 2 3 4 5 6 7 8 9 10 11 12

Fig. 8-53

ANALYSIS OF FIG. 8-53: Ventricular tachycardia is initially seen in Fig. 8-53. Following two fusion beats (6 and 7) and two supraventricular beats (8 and 9), ventricular tachycardia resumes and rapidly degenerates into ventricular fibrillation.

14. *Defibrillate* with 200 to 360 J of delivered energy.

Defibrillation results in the rhythm shown in Fig. 8-54. By this time you have made contact with the emergency physician at the nearest hospital. Transport of the patient is advised. What treatment would you institute en route for the rhythm shown in Fig. 8-54?

ANALYSIS OF FIG. 8-54: Following four agonal complexes, *asystole* results.

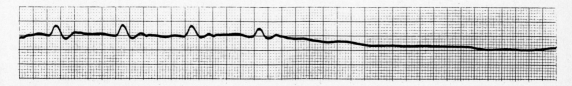

Fig. 8-54

15. Resume CPR.
16. Administer 2 ampules of *sodium bicarbonate*. (Considering the amount of time it took to establish an IV line, it is likely that significant metabolic acidosis has developed.)
17. Administer 1 mg of *epinephrine* IV. Be prepared to repeat this drug if the initial dose is not effective.
18. Consider administering 1 mg of *atropine*. (One milligram has already been given via the intratracheal route.)

19. Consider administering 500 mg of *calcium chloride* (5 ml of a 10% solution) IV.
20. Advise the emergency department that pacemaker insertion may be necessary on arrival.

On arrival in the emergency department the rhythm in Fig. 8-55 is observed. What is your interpretation?

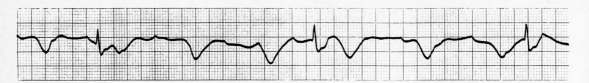

Fig. 8-55

ANALYSIS OF FIG. 8-55: An escape rhythm at a rate of about 20 beats/min is evident. Since the QRS configuration is identical to that seen in the supraventricular rhythms of previous tracings, the escape focus arises either from the AV node or the bundle of His. The wide negative deflections reflect ongoing CPR.

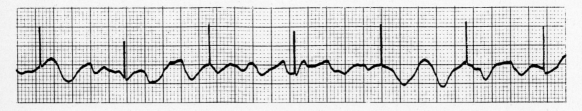

Fig. 8-56

A *transvenous pacemaker* is rapidly inserted by the emergency physician. Pacemaker spikes are evident in Fig. 8-56. Do you see anything else in this rhythm strip? What treatment is indicated?

ANALYSIS OF FIG. 8-56: The baseline of Fig. 8-56 is grossly irregular because of the presence of underlying ventricular fibrillation.

21. Defibrillate with 200 to 360 J.

Fig. 8-57 shows the result of defibrillation. Is the pacemaker functioning? What is the patient's underlying rhythm?

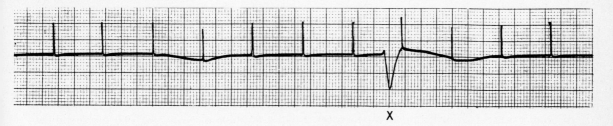

X

Fig. 8-57

ANALYSIS OF FIG. 8-57: Pacemaker spikes are seen at a rate of 90/min, but none of these are able to capture the ventricles. The only evidence of spontaneous activity is a single agonal complex (X).

The pacemaker wire is repositioned several times, but no ventricular capture can be obtained. Additional epinephrine, sodium bicarbonate, and calcium chloride are tried but to no avail. Resuscitative efforts are finally terminated.

Discussion

This patient succumbed to unexpected death of cardiac etiology within an hour of the onset of symptoms and therefore qualifies as a victim of *sudden cardiac death (SCD)*. This syndrome has become the single most common cause of death in the United States today, accounting for over 400,000 lives lost annually.

The initial mechanism of this patient's arrest was ventricular fibrillation. In communities with a well-developed EMS, on-the-scene resuscitation of ventricular fibrillation is successful in up to 60% of cases. About half of these patients survive to leave the hospital. The chances for immediate resuscitation are increased when the arrest is witnessed by an alert bystander who notifies the EMS and begins CPR. Ultimate sur-

vival with return to normal neurologic function is favored if the mobile rescue unit can then arrive within minutes to administer advanced life support.

The outcome of patients suffering from SCD has been shown to be directly related to the initial mechanism of arrest documented by the paramedic team on its arrival. Statistically, about two thirds of patients with cardiopulmonary arrest are initially found in ventricular fibrillation. An additional 5% to 10% are found in ventricular tachycardia with the remainder in a bradydysrhythmia (including asystole). Prognosis is best for those patients with ventricular tachycardia, the majority of whom undergo successful cardioversion. On the other hand, patients initially found in a bradydysrhythmia or asystole have a dismal prognosis with a virtual zero ultimate survival rate. The outcome of patients initially in ventricular fibrillation is intermediate between these two groups.

The initial documented mechanism of SCD may depend on the time between the onset of cardiovascular collapse and the time the paramedic team arrives. Thus it is likely that at least some cases of bradydysrhythmia represent a secondary rather than primary rhythm that succeeds ventricular fibrillation as time elapses.

The poor prognostic implications of brady-dysrhythmias carry over into the period immediately following resuscitation. For patients initially found in ventricular fibrillation, conversion to a rhythm with a heart rate greater than 100 beats/min (regardless of whether the rhythm is supraventricular or ventricular tachycardia) is associated with much better long-term survival rates than if the rhythm immediately following resuscitation is a bradydysrhythmia. Patients in whom the heart rate immediately after conversion from ventricular fibrillation is between 60 and 100 beats/min have an intermediate prognosis.

In the case study just presented, initial resuscitation of the patient from ventricular fibrillation was successful because of recognition of cardiopulmonary arrest by the son who started CPR and activated the EMS. The patient was rapidly defibrillated, but the immediate postconversion rhythm was a bradydysrhythmia. Subsequent development of asystole proved resistant to even the aggressive resuscitative effort that was attempted.

An awareness of the events leading to cardiac arrest, including all of the factors just mentioned, may provide the rescuer with important prognostic information regarding the chances of successful resuscitation and ultimate survival. This is not to say that little attempt should be made to resuscitate a patient in asystole who suffers an unwitnessed arrest but rather that knowledge of the clinical context in which the arrest occurs in conjunction with pertinent clinical information (knowledge of whether the patient has a terminal disease, etc.) may assist the rescuer in deciding if and when resuscitation efforts should be suspended. In the absence of such knowledge, the rescuer is obliged to continue CPR and advanced life support until it becomes evident that effective cardiovascular function cannot be restored.

NOTE: Case studies 9 through 13 are more advanced than the first 8 case studies and go a bit beyond the core content of most advanced life support courses.

CASE STUDY 9

A 68-year-old woman is admitted to the telemetry unit for a syncopal episode of unknown etiology. She is initially in sinus rhythm, but you are called to her room when she develops the rhythm shown in Fig. 8-58. She is alert, anxious, and complaining of "flut-tering" in her chest. Her blood pressure is 130/90 mm Hg. She does not have a heart murmur, but you hear loud bilateral carotid bruits. The patient is on no medications. What might this rhythm be? How would you proceed diagnostically and/or therapeutically?

Lead MCL₁

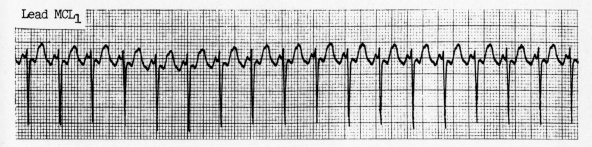

Fig. 8-58 Grauer, K., and Curry, R.W., Jr.: Monograph 47, AAFP Home Study Self-Assessment, © 1983, American Academy of Family Physicians.

ANALYSIS OF FIG. 8-58: There is a regular supraventricular tachycardia with a ventricular response of 150 beats/min. Normal sinus P waves are not evident. Although sinus tachycardia and PSVT should be included among the diagnostic possibilities, *the finding of a regular supraventricular tachycardia with a ventricular response of about 150 beats/min should strongly suggest atrial flutter with a 2:1 AV response.* The arrows in Fig. 8-59 indicate the flutter waves at a rate of 300 beats/min. Flutter waves can often be more clearly brought out by CSM, but this maneu-ver is risky in an elderly patient with carotid bruits, especially in one with syncope. Therapeutically, one might at this point do the following:

1. Have the patient perform a *Valsalva maneuver.*

   and/or

2. Administer 5 to 10 mg of *verapamil* IV (0.075 to 0.150 mg/kg) over a 1- to 4-minute period.

   and/or

3. *Digitalize* the patient.

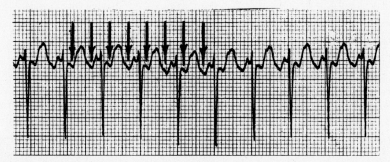

Fig. 8-59 Grauer, K., and Curry, R.W., Jr.: Monograph 47, AAFP Home Study Self-Assessment, © 1983, American Academy of Family Physicians.

Although atrial flutter is usually responsive to synchronized cardioversion at low energy levels, a trial of medical therapy would be appropriate in a patient who is tolerating the dysrhythmia.

Intravenous verapamil has become the drug of choice for treatment of PSVT, successfully converting this dysrhythmia over 90% of the time. In atrial fibrillation or atrial flutter, the use of verapamil is less likely to result in conversion to sinus rhythm, but the ventricular response is often significantly slowed. The half-life of an IV bolus of verapamil is relatively short, and the dose may need to be repeated at frequent intervals.

The patient is treated with a 0.5 mg IV bolus of *digoxin*. Shortly thereafter the rhythm in Fig. 8-60 is observed. What has happened?

Lead MCL$_1$

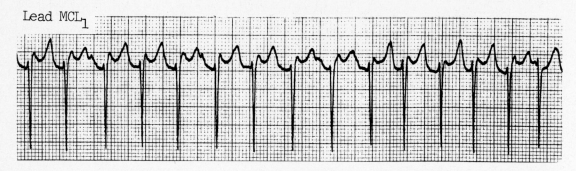

Fig. 8-60

ANALYSIS OF FIG. 8-60: Once again there is a rapid supraventricular tachycardia, but on close inspection the rhythm is now seen to be irregular. There is no identifiable atrial activity. This is *atrial fibrillation* with a *rapid ventricular response*, a diagnosis that could be easily overlooked unless one took the trouble to establish the irregular irregularity of the ventricular response. Atrial flutter usually does not become a chronic stable rhythm and often converts to atrial fibrillation.

A run of anomalous beats is observed a moment later (Fig. 8-61). A nurse asks if you want to give lidocaine?

Lead MCL$_1$

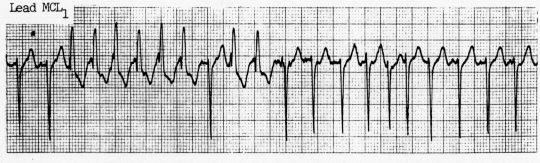

1 2 3 4 5 6 7 8 9 10 11 12 13 14 15 16 17 18 19 20 21

Fig. 8-61

ANALYSIS OF FIG. 8-61: The temptation is to call beats 3 to 8 a run of ventricular tachycardia. However, the morphology of these beats plus 10 and 11 demonstrates two of the principal features of aberrancy: an identical initial deflection to that of the normally conducted beats (upward in this case) and an RBBB pattern in a right-sided monitoring lead. Statistically, when runs of anomalous beats complicate rapid atrial fibrillation, they are more likely to be aberrantly conducted than PVCs. In addition, the irregular irregularity of the underlying rhythm continues throughout this run of anomalous beats. The run ends as abruptly as it begins, and there is no postectopic pause after beats 8 or 10. Taken together, the sum of these factors strongly favors *aberrancy*, and one would do better to withhold the lidocaine.

Two hours later, after an additional 0.25 mg of digoxin has been given, the rhythm in Fig. 8-62 is observed. Does this support your previous assumption that the anomalous beats in Fig. 8-61 were aberrant?

ANALYSIS OF FIG. 8-62: Sinus rhythm is temporarily restored (beats 1, 2, 3, and 5), but the rhythm then reverts back to atrial fibrillation. Beat 4 can be clearly identified as a PAC. This complex conducts normally, and a premature P wave distorts the preceding T wave. Similarly, a premature P wave produces a notch in the T wave preceding beat 6. Note that the morphology of beats 6, 7, 13, and 14 in Fig. 8-62 is identical to beats 3 to 8 and 10 and 11 of Fig. 8-61. In the context of Fig. 8-62, the premature P wave that precedes beat 6 in conjunction with the similar initial deflection to the normally conducted beats and an RBBB pattern establish beyond doubt that beat 6 is aberrantly conducted. It follows that all of the other similar appearing beats in this figure and Fig. 8-61 must also be aberrant. The reason beat 6 in Fig. 8-62 is conducted aberrantly and beat 4 (with an even shorter coupling interval) is not may be the result of the *Ashman phenomenon;* that is, the aberrant beat (6) follows the longest pause (the R-R interval between beats 4 and 5 is longer than that between beats 2 and 3).

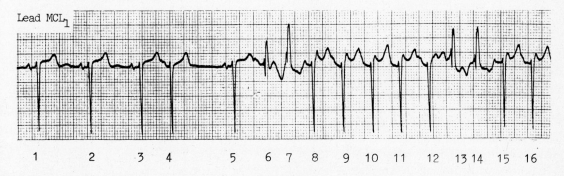

Fig. 8-62

A nurse now informs you that a run of anomalous beats manifesting still a different QRS configuration has just occurred (beats 13 to 16 in Fig. 8-63). She asks you if you want to give that lidocaine now?

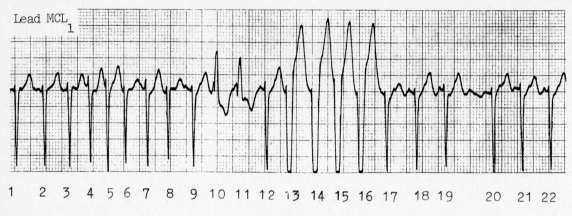

Fig. 8-63

ANALYSIS OF FIG. 8-63: Once again the underlying rhythm is atrial fibrillation with a rapid ventricular response. Beats 10 and 11 are recognized as being aberrantly conducted with an RBBB pattern. Their QRS configuration is identical to that of the anomalous beats just discussed.

Does beat 13 initiate a short run of ventricular tachycardia?

ANALYSIS: Beats 13 to 16 in Fig. 8-63 do not manifest an RBBB pattern, and the presence of atrial fibrillation precludes searching for telltale premature P waves. However, several other features suggest that these beats are also aberrantly conducted, this time with an LBBB pattern of aberrancy. First, note that the underlying irregular irregularity continues unabated throughout the entire rhythm strip in Fig. 8-63 and that the runs of anomalous beats again end as abruptly as they begin. Also note that the QRS duration of beats 13 to 16 is not greatly prolonged. Anomalous beats with a QRS duration of ≤ 0.12 are more likely to be aberrant than ectopic ventricular beats.

Finally, it is not generally appreciated that both RBBB and LBBB aberration commonly alternate in the same patient. This phenomenon of alternating RBBB and LBBB aberration should be particularly suspected when runs of anomalous beats are separated by a single normally conducted beat as they are by beat 12 in Fig. 8-63. Thus once again it would be better to withhold the lidocaine.

RBBB aberration occurs more frequently than LBBB aberration. Because of its characteristic morphology (it produces an rSR' in a right-sided monitoring lead), differentiation from ventricular ectopy usually does not pose much of a problem.

LBBB aberration may be far more difficult to recognize. It produces an rS or QS complex in a right-sided monitoring lead that often cannot be distinguished from a right ventricular PVC unless telltale features such as clearly identifiable premature P waves are seen (Fig. 6-13 on p. 86) or an irregular irregularity of the anomalous beats exists in the presence of underlying atrial fibrillation (Fig. 8-63).

This patient received two additional 0.25 mg increments of IV digoxin over the next 6 hours. Shortly thereafter the rhythm shown in Fig. 8-64 was recorded. By the next morning the patient was asymptomatic and in normal sinus rhythm (Fig. 8-65).

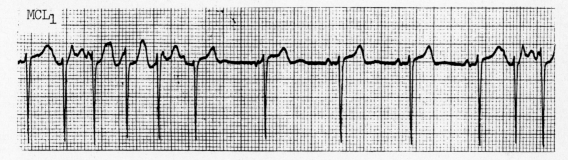

Fig. 8-64

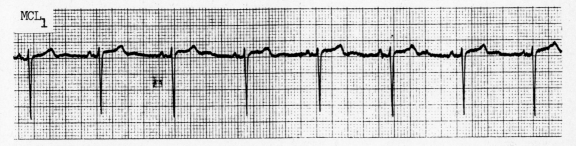

Fig. 8-65

Discussion

This case study emphasizes the importance of being able to differentiate PVCs from aberrantly conducted beats. Failure to do so would have resulted in mistreatment of the patient with lidocaine when what was needed to eliminate the anomalous beats was rather to treat the underlying primary disorder (rapid atrial fibrillation) that generated them.

Two additional factors to consider when contemplating whether or not anomalous beats may be aberrantly conducted are the following:

• Asking oneself if a reason exists for aberrancy

• Looking for the Ashman phenomenon

Aberrant conduction tends to be observed when a PAC or PJC occurs during the RRP. It is during this time that a portion of the conduction system (usually the right bundle branch) has not yet completely recovered. For example, if a premature impulse arrives at the bundle of His to find that the left bundle branch has totally recovered while the right bundle branch is still in a refractory state, the premature impulse will most likely be conducted with an RBBB pattern of aberration. The more refractory the premature impulse finds the ventricular conduction system (i.e., the earlier during the RRP that it occurs), the more likely it is that the beat will be conducted with aberration. Anomalous beats that occur after the RRP (i.e., anomalous beats that have a long coupling interval) have no reason to conduct aberrantly, since the conduction system will have had time to completely recover.

Examine Fig. 8-66. Are beats 2, 4, 6, and 8 PVCs, or are they aberrantly conducted?

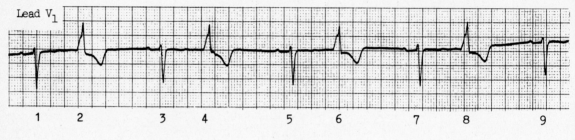

Fig. 8-66

ANALYSIS OF FIG. 8-66: Although the anomalous (even-numbered) beats in Fig. 8-66 manifest a similar initial deflection (upward) to the sinus conducted beats, they are wide and bizarre and have an oppositely directed T wave. They are not preceded by premature P waves. The fact that Fig. 8-66 is taken from a right-sided monitoring lead is of no assistance in the differentiation, since the r-slur-R' configuration is just as likely to be ectopic ventricular as it is to be aberrant (see Table 5-1 on p. 73). Finally, there is no reason for the even-numbered beats to conduct aberrantly, since they occur relatively late in the cycle (they have a long coupling interval) at a time when one would expect the entire conduction system to have completely recovered.

Recognition of the Ashman phenomenon may at times be helpful in differentiating PVCs from aberrancy. Simply stated, the Ashman phenomenon says that the most aberrant beat tends to follow the longest pause. This is because of the fact that the duration of the refractory period is proportional to the preceding R-R interval. In Fig. 8-62 the first anomalous beat (6) follows the longest pause in the rhythm strip (the R-R interval between beats 4 and 5). As a result, the refractory period of beat 5 is likely to be prolonged. Thus beat 6 has a "reason" for conducting aberrantly in that it probably occurs at a time when a portion of the conduction system (in this case the right bundle branch) is still refractory. (See Fig. 5-7 on p. 68.)

The coupling interval of premature beat 4 is even shorter than that of premature beat 6. Is there a reason beat 6 should conduct aberrantly, whereas beat 4 does not?

ANALYSIS: A possible reason beat 4 does not also conduct aberrantly is that its preceding R-R interval (the R-R between beats 2 and 3) is shorter than the R-R interval between beats 4 and 5 that precedes beat 6. Thus beat 6 conducts aberrantly by the Ashman phenomenon.

CASE STUDY 10

A 60-year-old man comes to the emergency department following a syncopal episode. The patient has a long history of coronary artery disease and ventricular dysrhythmias for which he is being treated with propranolol, long-acting nitrates, and procainamide. Fig. 8-67, taken from his old records, shows his most recent ECG.

On arrival in the emergency department the patient is anxious and complaining of palpitations. His blood pressure is 100/70 mm Hg, and he is in the rhythm shown in Fig. 8-68. How would you interpret this tracing?

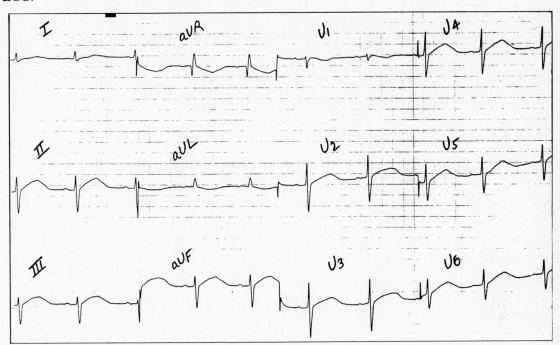

Fig. 8-67

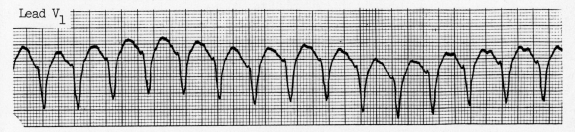

Fig. 8-68

ANALYSIS OF FIG. 8-68: There is a fairly regular tachydysrhythmia at a rate of about 135 beats/min. The QRS complex appears somewhat widened, and at first glance P waves are not evident, suggesting the possibility of ventricular tachycardia. As the heart rate slows ever so slightly for the last three beats of the strip, P waves can be seen to emerge from the ST segment (Fig. 8-69). This is *sinus tachycardia*.

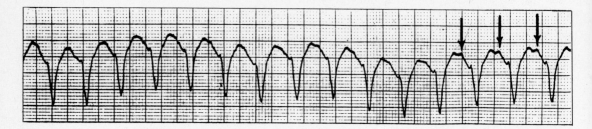

Fig. 8-69

Shortly thereafter the pulse weakens, and the rhythm shown in Fig. 8-70 is seen on the monitor. What is the rhythm? How would you treat this?

ANALYSIS OF FIG. 8-70: This is ventricular tachycardia.

1. Administer a *precordial thump*, since the onset of ventricular tachycardia was monitored.

and/or

2. Immediately use *cardioversion* on the patient with 200 J of delivered energy.

The patient's blood pressure is restored following cardioversion as he goes into the rhythm shown in Fig. 8-71. How would you interpret this tracing?

Lead V$_1$

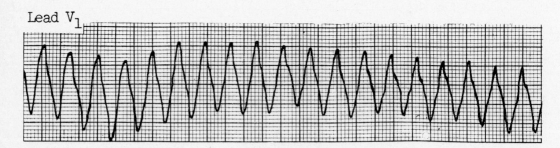

Fig. 8-70

ANALYSIS OF FIG. 8-71: Sinus tachycardia is present for beats 1 to 7 in Fig. 8-71. The P waves are again initially hidden but become more evident in front of beats 5 to 7 as the rate slows down. Beats 9 to 12 represent a short run of ventricular tachycardia. Beat 8 demonstrates a QRS configuration intermediate to the predominantly negative deflection of beats 1 to 7 and the positive deflection of the ventricular ectopic beats. This is a *fusion beat*.

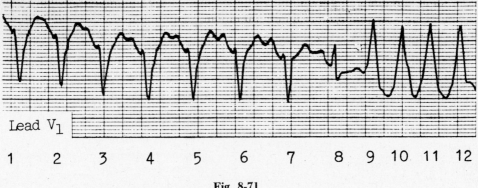

Lead V_1

1 2 3 4 5 6 7 8 9 10 11 12

Fig. 8-71

From beat 12 of Fig. 8-71 the patient goes into the rhythm shown in Figs. 8-72 and 8-73. What has happened? Would you give the patient more procainamide?

ANALYSIS OF FIGS. 8-72 AND 8-73: The rhythm deteriorates after beat 12 in Fig. 8-72. However, the polarity of the QRS complexes during the ventricular tachydysrhythmia alter-

nates from being predominantly positive (beats 10 to 16) to predominantly negative (beats 18 to 25). This changing polarity of ventricular tachycardia has been termed *torsade de pointes* (twisting of the points).

Originally described by the French physician Dessertenne in 1966, torsade de pointes often goes unrecognized and is mistreated as ordinary

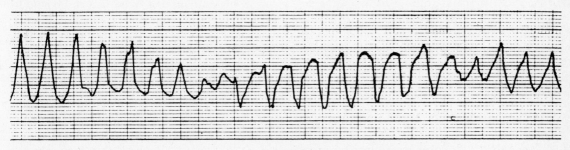

10 11 12 13 14 15 16 17 18 19 20 21 22 23 24 25

Fig. 8-72

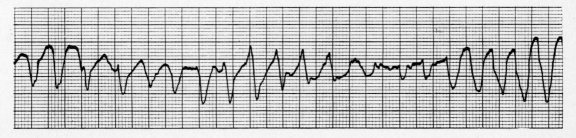

Fig. 8-73

ventricular tachycardia or ventricular fibrillation. This can have profound consequences for the patient who may be shocked countless times in an attempt to prevent this dysrhythmia from recurring. Drugs such as quinidine and procainamide that are usually effective in suppressing ventricular ectopy paradoxically exacerbate the dysrhythmia.

Torsade de pointes frequently is associated with a long QT interval on the baseline ECG. The dysrhythmia is thought to be triggered by the occurrence of a PVC at a relatively late point during the repolarization process. Paroxysms of ventricular tachycardia with alternating polarity ensue. These paroxysms often terminate spontaneously, but frequently recur until the underlying predisposing cause of QT prolongation has been corrected. Quinidine, disopyramide, and procainamide are absolutely contraindicated because these agents further prolong the QT interval.

The causes of torsade de pointes are essentially those of QT prolongation (box above at right). Of the antiarrhythmic drugs, quinidine is by far the most common precipitating agent. However, toxic levels of this drug need *not* be present for QT prolongation to occur, placing the onus on the physician to periodically check for QT prolongation.

CAUSES OF QT PROLONGATION AND TORSADE DE POINTES

Drugs
  Quinidine
  Procainamide
  Disopyramide
  Phenothiazines
  Tricyclic antidepressants
Electrolyte disturbances (i.e., hypokalemia)
Intrinsic heart disease
  Ischemic heart disease
  Myocarditis
Central nervous system catastrophe
  Subarachnoid hemorrhage
  Cerebrovascular accident
Liquid protein diet
Congenital QT prolongation syndrome

Since the best treatment of torsade de pointes lies in prevention, it is important to be able to recognize QT prolongation. Generally, the QT interval measures less than one half the R-R interval* (Fig. 8-74, A).

---

*This rule of thumb is less reliable for heart rates over 100 beats/min.

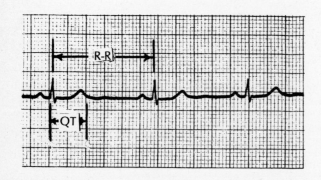

A

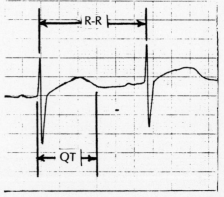

B

Fig. 8-74

Thus in Fig. 8-74, *B* the QT interval is prolonged. (Refer back to the 12-lead ECG shown in Fig. 8-67, and note that Fig. 8-74, *B* is taken from lead V_2 of this ECG.) The patient in this case study was being treated with procainamide, which should have been discontinued as soon as QT prolongation was recognized.

The goal of treatment of torsade de pointes is to eliminate predisposing factors when possible and to suppress the dysrhythmia until the QT interval returns to normal. It has already been discussed how drugs such as quinidine, disopyramide, and procainamide, which prolong the QT interval, are absolutely contraindicated in the treatment of this disorder. *Isoproterenol* shortens the QT interval and is recommended by many as the drug of choice. Use of this drug in the presence of rapid heart rates such as the one in Fig. 8-68 is controversial at best. Lidocaine and dilantin have little effect on the QT interval and have met with mixed success. *Cardioversion* may be required for prolonged episodes of torsade de pointes. More often than not this is only a temporary measure because of the dysrhythmia's disturbing tendency to recur. *Sequential overdrive pacing* is the generally accepted intervention of choice. Pacing at a rate of 80 to 120 beats/min usually allows control of the dysrhythmia until the precipitating factor is corrected and the QT interval comes back toward normal.

In this case overdrive pacing was used to control the patient's acute dysrhythmia; procainamide was withdrawn, and the QT interval gradually returned to normal.

CASE STUDY 11

A previously healthy 45-year-old man came to the emergency department with a 3-hour history of severe chest pain. Shortly after arrival the patient developed ventricular fibrillation, but prompt countershock with 200 J of delivered energy successfully converted him to sinus rhythm. His 12-lead ECG following conversion is shown in Fig. 8-75. How do you interpret this ECG?

ANALYSIS OF FIG. 8-75: Sinus tachycardia at a rate of about 100 beats/min is present. The QRS complex is widened, and there is complete RBBB. Q waves and ST-segment elevation in leads V_{1-4} suggest acute anterior infarction.

Does the patient need a pacemaker?

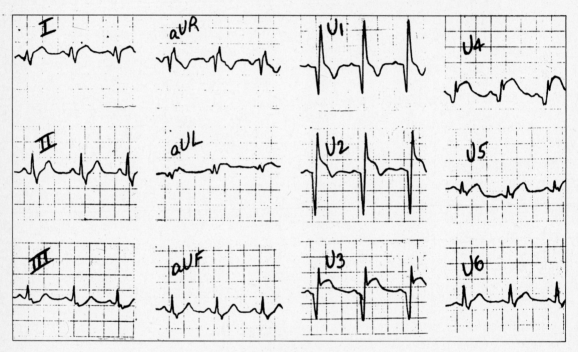

Fig. 8-75

ANALYSIS: The issue of when pacemaker insertion is indicated for conduction disturbances with acute myocardial infarction depends on the nature of the conduction defect and on the site of infarction. The ECG shown in Fig. 8-75 demonstrates a complete RBBB in the presence of acute anterior infarction. A critical question that cannot be answered on the basis of this tracing alone is whether the bundle branch block is new or old. If a previous ECG also demonstrated RBBB, insertion of a prophylactic pacemaker would probably not be necessary. One would be more concerned about progression to complete AV block if it were known for sure that the conduction disturbance was acute, but there is still disagreement regarding the need for prophylactic pacing with acute infarction and unifascicular block. Finally, if the block were bifascicular (i.e., RBBB and left anterior hemiblock, RBBB and left posterior hemiblock, alternating bundle branch block), there would be no question about the need for prophylactic pacemaker insertion.

Surprisingly, mortality in patients with acute anterior infarction and bifascicular block is linked not to the development of complete AV block but rather to development of cardiogenic shock. For this degree of impairment in the conduction system to take place, truly extensive myocardial damage must occur. Thus pacemaker insertion is indicated for the acute development of bifascicular bundle branch block in association with acute anterior infarction but probably does little to improve the dismal prognosis of these patients.

The cardiologist recommends that a pacemaker not be inserted. You are asked if you want to start the patient on prophylactic lidocaine?

ANALYSIS: Although caution must be advised in using lidocaine in the presence of intraventricular conduction disturbances such as the RBBB seen in this case, one must remember that the patient has already sustained one episode of ventricular fibrillation. The risk of recurrence almost certainly outweighs the risk posed by the careful administration of lidocaine to a patient with unifascicular bundle branch block.

1. Give the patient 75 to 100 mg IV bolus of *lidocaine*, and initiate a constant infusion to run at 2 mg/min.

Shortly after the lidocaine is infused, the patient regains consciousness. He complains of severe chest pain for which he is given several sublingual nitroglycerin tablets and a total of 10 mg of morphine sulfate IV. The chest pain continues. His lungs are clear, the neck veins are not distended, no murmur or gallop is heard on auscultation, and there is no peripheral edema. A chest x-ray film shows no signs of cardiac decompensation. Blood pressure is 160/100 mm Hg, and the patient's rhythm is shown in Fig. 8-76. Considering this overall picture, what would be the clinical significance of this rhythm?

ANALYSIS OF FIG. 8-76: The rhythm is *sinus tachycardia* at a rate of 110 beats/min. (Subtle P waves precede each QRS complex. There is borderline PR prolongation.)

Although the patient is not showing obvious clinical signs of cardiac decompensation, his rapid heart rate continues. Possible explanations for persistent tachycardia in the presence of acute infarction include the following:

Occult congestive heart failure. Studies with invasive hemodynamic monitoring have shown that up to 15% of patients with acute myocardial infarction have mild or moderate congestive heart failure with elevated pulmonary capillary wedge pressure (PCWP) that is not evident clinically.

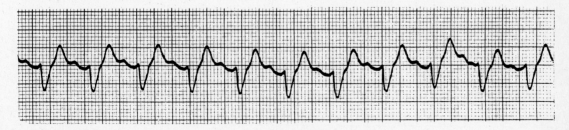

Fig. 8-76

Hypovolemia. With acute myocardial infarction, hypovolemia may be the result of inappropriate peripheral vasodilation.

Persistent chest pain. Chest pain and/or anxiety may cause sinus tachycardia. This patient's chest pain was not relieved, despite the liberal use of IV morphine sulfate and sublingual nitroglycerin.

Sympathetic hyperactivity. There is a high incidence of autonomic nervous system hyperactivity during the first hour of acute myocardial infarction. Parasympathetic hyperactivity with resultant sinus bradycardia and hypotension is particularly common with inferior infarction, whereas acute anterior infarction more often manifests sympathetic hyperactivity. Such sympathetic hyperactivity might account for the sinus tachycardia and hypertension seen in this patient.

In the presence of an acute infarction both sinus tachycardia and hypertension are deleterious because of the increased work load they place on the heart. Management of sinus tachycardia hinges on discovery and treatment of the underlying cause.

What would you do at this point?

ANALYSIS

2. Insert a Swan-Ganz catheter for diagnostic purposes and to assist with therapy. Indications for invasive hemodynamic monitoring in acute infarction are in the box on this page.

The pressure readings obtained from floating the flow-directed balloon-tipped catheter into the pulmonary capillary wedge position are as follows:

Right atrium—5 mm Hg (Normal = 0 to 8 mm Hg)

Right ventricle—36/7 mm Hg (Top normal = 30/8 mm Hg)

Pulmonary artery—36/23 mm Hg (Top normal = 30/12 mm Hg)

PCWP—25 mm Hg (Normal = 5 to 12 mm Hg)

INDICATIONS FOR INVASIVE HEMODYNAMIC MONITORING IN MYOCARDIAL INFARCTION

Persistent chest pain
Persistent tachycardia
Hypertension
Hypotension
Significant left ventricular failure
Use of intravenous nitroglycerin or nitroprusside for the management of any of the above
Development of a new systolic murmur (differentiation of ventricular septal defect from mitral regurgitation)

From Grauer, K.: Early management of myocardial infarction, Am. Fam. Physician **28**:166, 1983.

Cardiac index—2.1 L/min/m^2 (Normal = 2.5 L/min/m^2)

How do you interpret these readings? What treatment course would you follow for this patient?

ANALYSIS: The patient has relatively normal right-sided pressures, a significantly elevated PCWP, and a moderately depressed cardiac index. These readings are consistent with moderate congestive heart failure. Treatment might include the following:

3. Administer *diuretics* to decrease preload and reduce PCWP.

4. Give IV *nitroglycerin* to relieve the patient's persistent chest pain, treat his hypertension, and further reduce preload.

or

5. Administer IV *sodium nitroprusside* to improve cardiac output by reducing both preload and afterload as well as treating hypertension.

The patient is given 40 mg of *lasix* IV and is started on an infusion of IV nitroglycerin. This results in a 500 ml diuresis within an hour, a decrease in heart rate to 85 beats/min, disappearance of chest pain, and normalization of blood pressure. The cardiac index increases to 2.5 L/min/m^2 as the PCWP drops to 16 mm Hg. The patient recovers without further complications.

Discussion

Despite all of the therapeutic advancements made during the past decade, many patients with acute myocardial infarction still die of ventricular fibrillation while at home. This is because of the average 2- to 3-hour delay between the onset of symptoms and the time the patient decides to call for medical assistance. When one considers that by far the greatest danger of developing ventricular fibrillation with acute myocardial infarction is during the first 1 to 2 hours, it becomes easy to see why the majority of patients dying from acute myocardial infarction do so before they ever reach the hospital. This patient's story is typical. He stayed at home with chest pain for 3 hours before seeking medical assistance. Had he waited another 5 minutes before calling for an ambulance, he would have fibrillated at home and probably would not have survived. For further improvement in survival of patients with acute myocardial infarction to take place, additional efforts must be directed at teaching the public to recognize the signs and symptoms of acute myocardial infarction and calling for help promptly.

CASE STUDY 12

A 62-year-old woman is rushed to the emergency department following a syncopal episode. On arrival she is conscious, but her pulse is extremely rapid and thready. A blood pressure of only 90/60 mm Hg is recorded, and her rhythm is shown in Fig. 8-77. Is this ventricular tachycardia? Is it rapid atrial fibrillation?

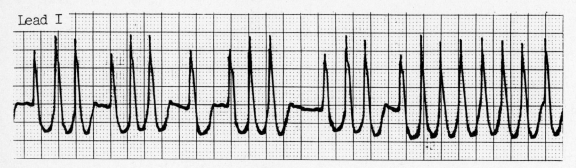

Fig. 8-77

ANALYSIS OF FIG. 8-77: Although the QRS duration varies in different parts of this tracing, most complexes are widened, and there is no atrial activity. However, the gross irregularity of this rhythm makes ventricular tachycardia highly unlikely. Ordinary atrial fibrillation is ruled out by the rapidity of the rate. In certain areas the R-R interval between QRS complexes is just over one large box in duration, which corresponds to a ventricular response of about 250 beats/min. This is too fast for atrial impulses to be transmitted to the ventricles by the normal conduction pathway, since the refractory period of the AV node will not allow so rapid a rate. The only reasonable explanation is that the atrial impulses are bypassing the AV node and are being conducted to the ventricles via an *accessory pathway* with a much shorter refractory period.

This patient's 12-lead ECG is shown in Fig. 8-78. Is the underlying diagnosis more evident?

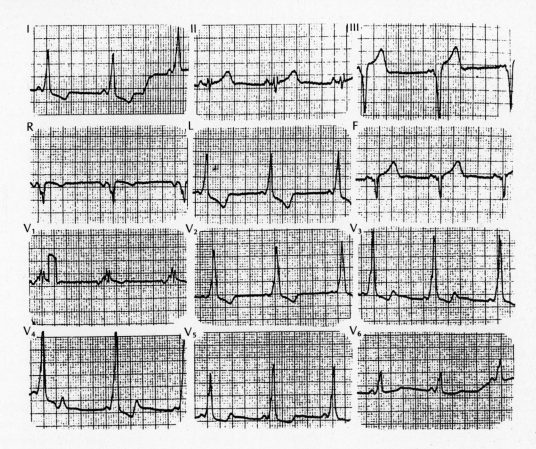

Fig. 8-78 Grauer, K., and Curry, R.W., Jr.: Monograph 47, AAFP Home Study Self-Assessment, © 1983, American Academy of Family Physicians.

ANALYSIS OF FIG. 8-78: The diagnosis of *Wolff-Parkinson-White (WPW) syndrome* is now obvious from the short PR interval, QRS widening, and slurring (delta waves) of the initial portions of the QRS complex.

WPW has an approximate incidence of two per every thousand individuals in the general population. Conduction of the sinus impulse may be via the normal AV nodal pathway, it may

be down the accessory tract, or it may alternate between the two. Patients with WPW are prone to develop atrial tachydysrhythmias in which a reentry circuit is set up between the normal AV nodal pathway and the accessory tract. With PSVT this most often results in antegrade conduction down the *AV nodal pathway* (producing a narrow QRS complex during the tachycardia) and retrograde conduction via the accessory pathway (Fig. 8-79, A). This tachydysrhythmia is

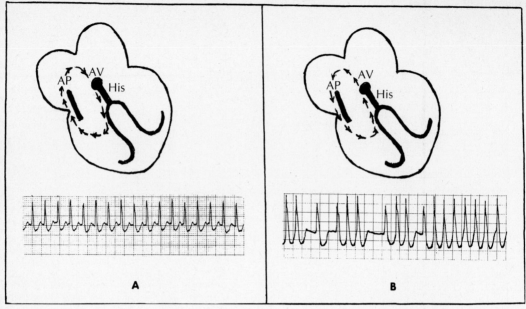

Fig. 8-79

AP - Accessory Pathway
AV - AV Nodal Pathway
His - Bundle of His

usually well tolerated by the patient.

In contrast, with atrial fibrillation in WPW, antegrade conduction usually occurs down the *accessory tract* with retrograde conduction to the AV nodal pathway. This results in QRS widening during the tachycardia. Because of the short refractory period of the accessory pathway, there may be 1:1 conduction of atrial impulses during atrial fibrillation, resulting in a ventricular response that exceeds 250 beats/min (Fig. 8-79, *B*). Such rapid rates may not be well tolerated, and this rhythm can deteriorate into ventricular fibrillation. Similarly, antegrade conduction down the accessory pathway frequently occurs when patients with WPW develop atrial flutter, resulting in a ventricular response that may exceed 300 beats/min.

Now return to Fig. 8-77. Would you treat this patient with IV digoxin in an attempt to slow the ventricular response?

ANALYSIS: Although IV digoxin is extremely effective in slowing the ventricular rate in ordinary atrial fibrillation with a rapid ventricular response, it is contraindicated in WPW with atrial fibrillation. This is because *digoxin may further accelerate conduction down the accessory pathway and exacerbate the dysrhythmia.*

The patient was nevertheless given 0.5 mg of IV digoxin. Shortly thereafter the rhythm in Fig. 8-77 deteriorated to that shown in Fig. 8-80. What has happened? What would you do at this point?

ANALYSIS OF FIG. 8-80: Digoxin probably accelerated conduction down the accessory pathway leading to an increase in the rate of the atrial fibrillation and development of ventricular fibrillation.

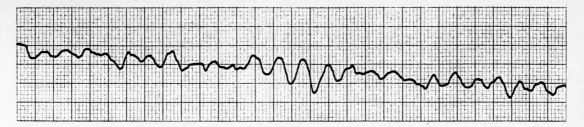

Fig. 8-80

1. Defibrillate the patient with 200 J of delivered energy.

Defibrillation results in a reversion of the rhythm to the rapid atrial fibrillation (Fig. 8-81). Realizing that digoxin only made things worse, is there any other medical therapy that you might offer this patient?

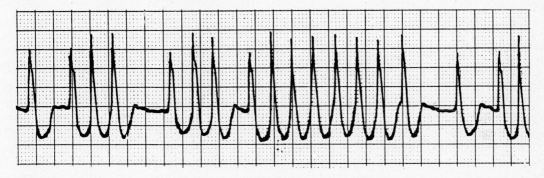

Fig. 8-81

ANALYSIS OF FIG. 8-81: The goal of treating rapid atrial fibrillation with WPW is to prevent the 1:1 antegrade conduction of atrial impulses down the accessory pathway. This can be done by lengthening the antegrade refractory period of the accessory pathway, an effect shared by procainamide and lidocaine:

2. Give the patient a loading dose of 10 mg/kg of *procainamide* IV in 100 mg increments or slow intravenous infusion over 30 minutes.

or

3. Administer an initial bolus of 75 to 100 mg of *lidocaine* followed by several additional 50 to 75 mg boluses at 5-minute intervals.

The rhythm in Fig. 8-81 is treated with IV procainamide. A total of 500 mg has been given when a sigh of relief is heard throughout the room. The monitor now reflects the rhythm shown in Fig. 8-82.

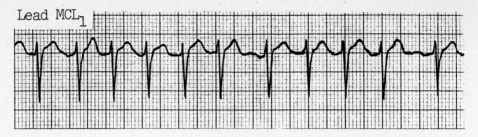

Lead MCL_1

Fig. 8-82

ANALYSIS OF FIG. 8-82: Atrial fibrillation is still present, but the ventricular response—although still rapid—is much slower than it was in Fig. 8-81, and the QRS complex is now of normal duration. By blocking antegrade conduction down the accessory pathway, atrial impulses can now be transmitted via the AV nodal pathway. As a result, the QRS complex is narrow, and the ventricular response to the atrial fibrillation is controlled.

Discussion

When confronted with a wide-complex tachy-dysrhythmia that is grossly irregular yet registers a rate of over 220 beats/min, WPW should be assumed until proven otherwise. Supraventricular impulses with ordinary atrial fibrillation cannot be conducted down the AV nodal pathway at so rapid a rate. Similarly, ventricular tachycardia rarely occurs at such rapidity or with that degree of irregularity. Whereas giving a patient a loading dose of IV digoxin is effective in controlling the ventricular response of ordinary atrial fibrillation, the drug may have the opposite effect when used in the presence of an accessory pathway. In addition to potentially acceler-ating conduction of atrial impulses down the accessory pathway, the use of digoxin also makes any subsequent attempts at electrical cardioversion more hazardous. On the other hand, the use of digoxin is probably safe in patients with WPW and PSVT with a narrow QRS complex (antegrade conduction down the normal AV nodal pathway [Fig. 8-79, A]).

Remarkable for its absence in the discussion of this case is verapamil. This drug has an unpredictable effect on the refractory period of the accessory pathway and consequently, should probably *not* be used to treat rapid atrial fibrillation with WPW. On the other hand, verapamil lengthens the refractory period of the AV nodal pathway and is the drug of choice for treating PSVT when the QRS complex is narrow during the tachydysrhythmia, regardless of whether or not the patient has WPW.

Although the incidence of WPW in the general population is not high, it occurs frequently enough that the emergency care provider probably will encounter several cases during his or her career. An awareness of this syndrome and the potentially disastrous consequences that may ensue if rapid atrial fibrillation develops may therefore prove invaluable.

CASE STUDY 13

You are working in a rural clinic where a 47-year-old man comes in with a 1-hour history of severe chest pain. He is diaphoretic and has a blood pressure of 90/70 mm Hg at the time the 12-lead ECG shown in Fig. 8-83 is taken. How do you interpret this tracing?

ANALYSIS OF FIG. 8-83: There is a bradydysrhythmia present with a narrow complex ventricular response at about 48 beats/min. The PR intervals appear to vary in the different leads, indicating AV dissociation. The ST-segment elevation in leads II, III, and aVF with reciprocal ST-segment depression in the anterolateral leads in conjunction with the history suggest *acute inferior infarction*.

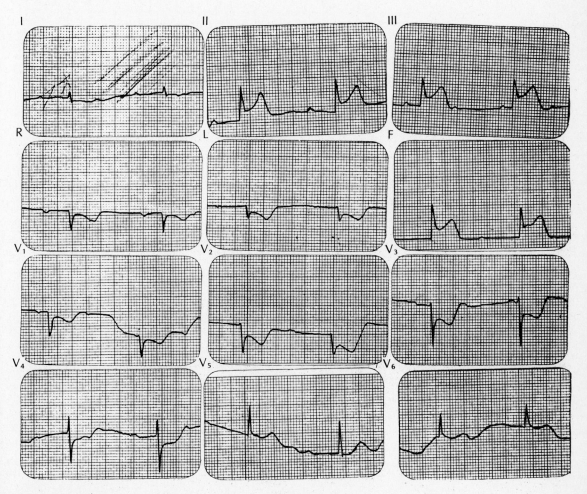

Fig. 8-83

Does the rhythm strip shown in Fig. 8-84 help you to determine the rhythm?

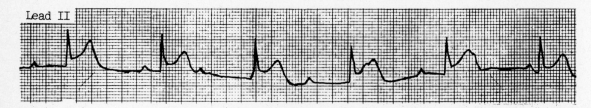

Fig. 8-84

ANALYSIS OF FIG. 8-84: The atrial rate is now regular at 80 beats/min, and P waves march through the QRS complexes (Fig. 8-85). This is *third-degree AV block* with a junctional escape pacemaker.

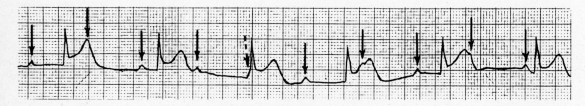

Fig. 8-85

The patient's lungs are clear to auscultation, and a chest x-ray film does not suggest pulmonary congestion. There is no jugular venous distention or peripheral edema. Considering that facilities for pacemaker insertion are not available in this clinic and that the nearest hospital is over an hour away, how would you treat the patient?

ANALYSIS
1. Start an IV line with D_5W.
2. Give supplemental *oxygen* by nasal cannula.
3. Administer *atropine* 0.5 mg IV. Be prepared to follow this with additional 0.5 mg increments if there is no improvement in the ventricular response.
4. Medicate the patient with *sublingual nitroglycerin* and/or *morphine sulfate* 3 to 5 mg IV every 5 to 10 minutes as needed.
5. Consider the use of prophylactic *lidocaine*.

Atropine sulfate is the medical treatment of choice for a symptomatic bradydysrhythmia in the presence of acute infarction. This is particularly true when the infarction is inferior and the rhythm may be the result of excessive parasympathetic tone or ischemia of the AV node rather than an irreversible anatomic defect in the conduction system. In many such instances AV block even if complete is short-lived, may respond to atropine, and does not require pacemaker insertion if an adequate escape focus exists. In this case the decision of whether or not a pacemaker should be inserted is academic, since it will be at least an hour before you come into contact with a physician capable of inserting one.

Nitroglycerin and morphine sulfate are recommended for treating chest pain in the presence of acute ischemia, but they should be used cautiously when the patient is hypotensive.

Morphine may sometimes cause bradycardia. Despite the presence of complete AV block, lidocaine prophylaxis should be considered because of the high risk of developing primary ventricular fibrillation during the first few hours of acute infarction.

The patient is given 3 mg of morphine sulfate IV and two 0.5 mg doses of atropine. His blood pressure has now increased to 110/70 mm Hg, his chest pain is less, and he is in the rhythm shown in Fig. 8-86. What is this rhythm?

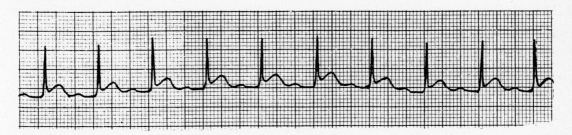

Fig. 8-86

ANALYSIS OF FIG. 8-86: The sinus rate has increased to 105 beats/min, and there is now 1:1 AV conduction (sinus rhythm) with first-degree AV block.

Over the next 2 minutes the patient successively develops the rhythms shown in Fig. 8-87 to 8-89. His blood pressure drops to 80/60 mm Hg. What has happened? What would you do?

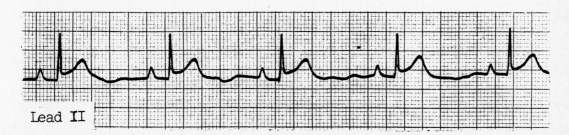

Lead II

Fig. 8-87

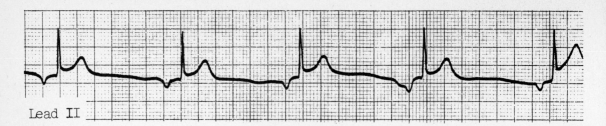

Lead II

Fig. 8-88

ANALYSIS OF FIGS. 8-87 TO 8-89: The sinus rate in Fig. 8-87 has slowed to 50 beats/min. In Fig. 8-88 there has been further slowing of the ventricular response to 43 beats/min with a shift in the atrial pacemaker to a low atrial focus (evidenced by the negative P wave in lead II). Finally, in Fig. 8-89 the P wave has disappeared with the onset of junctional rhythm, and the ventricular response has slowed to 38 beats/min. Thus the site of impulse formation has moved progressively more distal in the conduction system.

6. Elevate the foot of the bed.
7. Administer additional 0.5 mg increments of *atropine* until a total of 2 mg has been given.

If both of these measures fail to correct the hypotension, what might you try?

ANALYSIS
8. Cautiously attempt *fluid challenge*, infusing 100 ml increments of D_5W or normal saline solution.
                    and/or
9. Try an infusion of either *dopamine, isoproterenol,* or *epinephrine*.

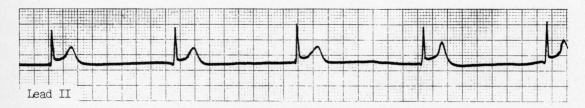

Lead II

Fig. 8-89

With the administration of an additional 1 mg of atropine the patient's blood pressure returns to 105/70 mm Hg, and his rhythm develops into that shown in Fig. 8-90. What has happened? Is further treatment indicated?

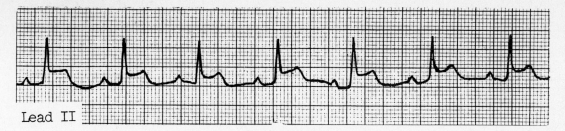

Lead II

Fig. 8-90

ANALYSIS OF FIG. 8-90: There is now sinus rhythm at 70 beats/min with borderline first-degree AV block. The patient's condition has stabilized, and transport to the nearest hospital may be undertaken.

Discussion

Bradydysrhythmias and hypotension are frequent accompaniments of acute inferior infarction. These effects often result from the parasympathetic overactivity that occurs during the early hours of the infarction, and they commonly respond to treatment with atropine. Hypotension with acute infarction may also be the result of relative hypovolemia caused by inappropriate peripheral vasodilation or the absolute hypovolemia from fluid depletion (dehydration, improper use of diuretics with acute infarction). The heart rate is either normal or increased, and elevation of the lower extremities with cautious administration of volume is the treatment of choice. A rise in blood pressure with a fall in heart rate indicates a favorable response to volume replacement. The most ominous cause of hypotension with acute infarction is the onset of cardiogenic shock. In this case the pulse is rapid in the presence of pulmonary congestion and peripheral vasoconstriction, and the patient's condition is made worse by the administration of fluid. Definitive diagnosis is made by passage of a Swan-Ganz catheter.

In this case study both the bradycardia and hypotension responded to atropine, suggesting excessive vagotonia as the precipitating cause.

Suggested Readings
Case Study 8

Cobb, L.A., and Werner, J.A.: Predictors and prevention of sudden cardiac death. In Hurst, J.W., (editor): The heart, New York, 1982, McGraw-Hill Book Co., pp. 599-610.

Eisenberg, M., Hallstrom, A., and Bergner, L.: The ACLS score—predicting survival from out-of-hospital cardiac arrest, JAMA **246**:50-52, 1981.

Grauer, K.: Sudden cardiac death, Cont. Ed. **17**:82-86, 1983.

Myerburg, R.J., Kessler, K.M., Zaman, L., Conde, C.A., and Castellanos, A.: Survivors of prehospital cardiac arrest, JAMA **247**:1485-1490, 1982.

Case Study 9

Marriott, H.J.L., and Conover, M.H.B.: Advanced concepts in arrhythmias, St. Louis, 1983, The C.V. Mosby Co., pp. 244-267.

Case Study 10

Kemper, A.J., Dunlap, R., and Pietro, D.A.: Thioridazine-induced torsade de pointes: successful therapy with isoproterenol, JAMA **249**:2931-2934, 1983.

Kim, H.S., and Chung, E.K.: Torsade de pointes: polymorphous ventricular tachycardia, Heart Lung **12**:269-273, 1983.

Parrish, C., Wooster, W.E., Braen, G.R., and Robertson, H.D.: Les torsade de pointes, Ann. Emerg. Med. **11**:143-146, 1982.

Smith, W.M., and Gallagher, J.J.: Les torsades de pointes: an unusual ventricular arrhythmia, Ann. Intern. Med. **93**:578-584, 1980.

Case Study 11

Forrester, J.S., Diamond, G., Chatterjee, K., and Swan, H.J.C.: Medical therapy of acute myocardial infarction by application of hemodynamic subsets, Part 1, N. Engl. J. Med. **295**:1356-1362, 1976.

Forrester, J.S., Diamond, G., Chatterjee, K., and Swan, H.J.C.: Medical therapy of acute myocardial infarction by application of hemodynamic subsets, Part 2, N. Engl. J. Med. **295:**1404-1413, 1976.

Grauer, K.: Early management of myocardial infarction, Am. Fam. Physician **28:**162-170, 1983.

Hindman, M.C., Wagner, G.S., JaRo, M., Atkins, J.M., Scheinman, M.M., DeSanctis, R.W., Hutter, A.H., Yeatman, L., Rubenfire, M., Pujura, C., Rubin, M., and Morris, J.J.: The clinical significance of bundle branch block complicating acute myocardial infarction, Circulation **58:**679-699, 1978.

Loeb, H.S., and Gunnar, R.M.: Treatment of pump failure in acute myocardial infarction, JAMA **245:**2093-2096, 1981.

Scheinman, M.M., and Gonzalez, R.P.: Fascicular block and acute myocardial infarction, JAMA **244:**2646-2649, 1980.

Case Study 12

Chung, E.K.: Electrocardiography: practical applications with vectorial principles, New York, 1980, Harper & Row, Publishers, pp. 280-304.

Kuhn, M.: Verapamil in the treatment of PSVT, Ann. Emerg. Med. **10:**538-544, 1981.

PART FOUR

SELF-ASSESSMENT IN CARDIAC ARREST

SELF-ASSESSMENT IN CARDIAC ARREST

This section provides readers with an opportunity to assess their general knowledge in cardiac resuscitation and their ability in dysrhythmia interpretation. Areas of strength and weakness can thus be identified and a personalized study program formulated either for self-improvement and/or in preparation for a formal course in advanced life support.

Answers to the multiple choice and true or false questions have been referenced (to this book, the AHA *Textbook of Advanced Cardiac Life Support* (1981), and/or the *JAMA* supplement) to indicate where additional information may be found. Detailed answers to the dysrhythmia questions follow the rhythm strips. The reader is referred to Chapters 4 to 7 in Part II of this book for additional information on dysrhythmia interpretation.

GENERAL MANAGEMENT QUIZ

Choose the correct letter. Many questions have more than one correct answer.

1. Steps in the assessment and management of the unconscious victim include:
   1. Calling for help
   2. Establishing unresponsiveness
   3. Positioning the victim
   4. Applying the ABCs of CPR
   Which one of the following indicates the correct order in which these steps should be performed?
   A. 1,2,3,4
   B. 1,3,2,4
   C. 2,1,3,4
   D. 2,3,4,1
   E. 4,1,2,3
2. Treatment for asystole includes which of the following?
   A. Epinephrine
   B. Sodium bicarbonate
   C. Atropine
   D. Calcium chloride
   E. Pacemaker insertion
3. The single most common cause of airway obstruction in the unconscious victim is:

A. A foreign body
B. Food
C. Dentures
D. The tongue
E. Edema from epiglottitis or tracheobronchitis

4. For external chest compression to be effective in an adult, the sternum must be depressed:
   A. ½ to ¾ inch
   B. 1 inch
   C. 1½ to 2 inches
   D. 2½ inches
   E. 3 to 4 inches
5. Which of the following measures may be useful in the treatment of paroxysmal supraventricular tachycardia?
   A. Sedation
   B. Verapamil
   C. Carotid sinus massage
   D. Infusion of isoproterenol
   E. Digitalization
6. Which of the following factors are important in determining survival from out-of-hospital ventricular fibrillation?
   A. Prompt recognition of cardiac arrest by the lay public and early activation of emergency medical services
   B. Initiation of CPR by a bystander within 4 minutes
   C. Initiation of advanced life support within 8 minutes
   D. The mechanism of the arrest
   E. All of the above
7. Regarding the diagnosis of acute myocardial infarction, which one of the following is the most important factor to consider in deciding to admit a patient with chest pain?
   A. Initial ECG
   B. Chest x-ray film
   C. Cardiac enzymes
   D. Technetium pyrophosphate scan
   E. History
8. Which of the following statements is/are true regarding supraventricular bradydysrhythmias with acute myocardial infarction?
   A. They are particularly common during the first hour following the onset of symptoms.
   B. They are most often associated with anterior infarction.
   C. They usually reflect increased parasympathetic tone.
   D. They should be routinely treated with atropine.
   E. All of the above.

9. Which of the following statements is/are true regarding current recommendations for the performance of two-rescuer CPR?
   A. Sixty compressions should be performed each minute.
   B. There should be a 15:2 ventilation to compression ratio.
   C. Each compression should be sustained for 40% of the cycle.
   D. CPR may be stopped for up to 45 seconds at a time when needed for endotracheal intubation or moving a patient.
   E. The cardiac output produced by properly performed external chest compression may be 60% of normal output.

10. One establishes pulselessness in an infant by checking for the presence of:
    A. Carotid pulse
    B. Brachial pulse
    C. Radial pulse
    D. Precordial activity
    E. Femoral pulse

11. The most common mechanism of sudden cardiac death is:
    A. Ventricular tachycardia
    B. Ventricular fibrillation
    C. Asystole
    D. Electromechanical dissociation
    E. Long QT syndrome

12. In an unmonitored arrest situation, what should be done first once the diagnosis of ventricular fibrillation has been established?
    A. Deliver a precordial thump.
    B. Apply countershock with 200 to 300 J of delivered energy.
    C. Apply countershock with 360 J of delivered energy.
    D. Administer epinephrine IV or by intratracheal instillation.
    E. Administer sodium bicarbonate.

13. Which of the following statements about sodium bicarbonate is/are true?
    A. The initial dose for a patient in cardiac arrest is 1 mEq/kg.
    B. Additional doses of sodium bicarbonate are ideally governed by the results of ABGs.
    C. In the event that ABGs are not available, one half of the initial dose may be repeated every 5 minutes.
    D. It is probably unnecessary to give any sodium bicarbonate if the period of arrest is less than 1 minute.
    E. Each ampule of sodium bicarbonate contains 25 mEq of drug.

14. The recommended dose of epinephrine for IV administration is:
    A. 0.05 to 0.10 mg of a 1:10,000 solution
    B. 0.5 to 1.0 mg of a 1:10,000 solution
    C. 5 to 10 mg of a 1:10,000 solution
    D. 0.5 to 1.0 mg of a 1:1000 solution
    E. 5 to 10 mg of a 1:1000 solution

15. Clinical indications of lidocaine toxicity include which of the following?
    A. Disorientation
    B. Paresthesias
    C. Diarrhea
    D. Agitation
    E. Seizures

16. Which of the following statements about procainamide is/are true?
    A. The drug may be administered in 100 mg increments IV every minute until a loading dose of 1 g has been given.
    B. Its use is indicated for ventricular dysrhythmias that are resistent to lidocaine.
    C. Its use may widen the QRS complex.
    D. It may cause hypotension when given IV.
    E. The drug may cause atrioventricular conduction disturbance.

17. Which of the following statements about dopamine is/are true?
    A. The drug is a chemical precursor of norepinephrine.
    B. At doses above 20 μg/kg/min it dilates renal and mesenteric blood vessels.
    C. It primarily exerts an α-receptor stimulating action at low doses.
    D. It is indicated for treatment of cardiogenic shock and hemodynamically significant hypotension.
    E. It comes in 1 ml ampules that contain 500 mg of drug.

18. What would you expect the pH to be for a patient with a pure respiratory acidosis if the P_{aCO_2} is 55 torr?
    A. 7.36
    B. 7.32
    C. 7.28
    D. 7.24
    E. 7.20

19. Cannulation of the internal jugular vein by the central approach is performed by introducing the needle:
    A. 1 cm below the junction of the middle and medial thirds of the clavicle
    B. At the midpoint of the anterior border of the sternomastoid muscle
    C. At the junction of the lower and middle thirds of the anterior border of the sternomastoid muscle

D. At the apex of the triangle formed by the two heads of the sternomastoid muscle and the clavicle

E. Under the sternomastoid muscle near the junction of the middle and lower thirds of the lateral border of this muscle

20. Which of the following statements about airway obstruction is/are true?

A. Dentures and an elevated blood alcohol level are frequently associated with choking on food.

B. Foreign body obstruction of the airway accounts for nearly as many cases of cardiopulmonary arrest as does coronary heart disease.

C. Back blows and manual thrusts should be applied in the management of both partial and total airway obstruction.

D. Foreign body obstruction of the airway rarely occurs during eating.

E. The abdominal thrust to relieve airway obstruction cannot be applied by the victim on himself.

21. Which of the following statements is/are true regarding the performance of basic life support in infants and children?

A. Only two fingers are needed to perform adequate external chest compression in the infant.

B. The proper area of compression in the infant is the midsternum.

C. The sternum should be depressed ¼ to ½ inch with external chest compression in the infant.

D. The compression to ventilation ratio is 5:1 for one and two rescuers.

E. The compression rate in infants is 80/min.

22. What is the recommended initial energy dose for the defibrillation of a 20 kg child?

A. 10 J
B. 20 J
C. 40 J
D. 60 J
E. 80 J

23. Which of the following statements about the esophageal obturator airway is/are true?

A. It should only be used in unconscious patients.

B. It may be used in children over the age of 10 years.

C. It should not be used when esophageal disease is suspected.

D. Endotracheal intubation cannot be accomplished while the EOA is in place.

E. Inflation of the esophageal obturator airway cuff requires as much air as inflation of the cuff of an endotracheal tube.

24. The most common cause of sudden cardiac death is:

A. Mitral valve prolapse
B. Coronary heart disease

C. Acute myocardial infarction
D. Hypertrophic cardiomyopathy
E. Massive pulmonary thromboembolism

25. Which of the following statements about Mobitz I second-degree AV block is/are true?

A. This form of block usually occurs below the level of the AV node.

B. The conduction defect is usually transient.

C. The block may be the result of the increased parasympathetic tone that is commonly associated with acute inferior infarction.

D. Group beating is commonly seen.

E. The block may be caused by digitalis toxicity.

26. Which of the following statements about atrial flutter is/are true?

A. The atrial rate is usually about 300 beats/min.

B. The ventricular response is usually about 100 beats/min.

C. The rhythm is a common manifestation of digitalis toxicity.

D. The rhythm is usually easily converted to sinus rhythm with low energy cardioversion.

E. Application of carotid sinus massage may be helpful in confirming the diagnosis.

27. Which of the following factors would suggest that an abnormal QRS complex is an aberrantly conducted premature atrial contraction, rather than a premature ventricular contraction?

A. The finding of a premature P wave in front of the abnormal complex

B. The presence of a full compensatory pause

C. A QRS complex width of greater than 0.14 second for the abnormal complex

D. A right bundle branch block pattern of the abnormal complex in a right-sided monitoring lead

E. The presence of atrial fibrillation

28. Treatment for ventricular tachycardia may include which of the following?

A. Cardioversion
B. Lidocaine
C. Procainamide
D. Verapamil
E. Bretylium

29. Treatment for third-degree AV block may include which of the following?

A. Verapamil
B. Isoproterenol
C. Insertion of a pacemaker
D. Calcium chloride
E. Atropine

30. Insertion of a subclavian or internal jugular line is preferable on the right side because of which of the following reasons?
    A. The dome of the right lung and pleura is lower than it is on the left side.
    B. Both veins are larger on the right side.
    C. There is more or less a straight line to the atrium.
    D. The landmarks are easier to recognize on the right side.
    E. The large thoracic duct is not endangered.

Indicate whether questions 31 to 50 are true or false.

31. In the "sniffing" position the neck is extended backward as the head is flexed forward.
32. To intubate a patient with a curved blade, the tip is inserted into the vallecula, and traction is exerted upward and forward to displace the epiglottis anteriorly and expose the glottis.
33. The tidal volumes generated with a bag-valve-mask device are much greater than those delivered by the mouth-to-mouth technique.
34. A Venturi mask is advantageous for use in patients with chronic obstructive pulmonary disease because of its ability to deliver a controlled oxygen concentration.
35. The femoral vein lies medial to the artery in the femoral sheath.
36. Cardiac arrest in children is usually secondary to hypoxia produced by a respiratory arrest.
37. The most common adverse reaction to bretylium is hypertension.
38. Nitroglycerin is contraindicated in the management of acute myocardial infarction, since there is the risk of it causing hypotension.

39. Ventricular fibrillation is more than 10 times as common during the first 2 hours after the onset of symptoms of an acute myocardial infarction than during the subsequent 24 hours.
40. The Killip classification for patients with acute myocardial infarction can reliably predict which patients will have elevated pulmonary capillary wedge pressures with hemodynamic monitoring.
41. Induction of diuresis is the treatment of choice for right-sided heart failure associated with pure right ventricular infarction.
42. The insertion of a pacemaker has been conclusively shown to reduce mortality in patients who develop complete right bundle branch block with acute myocardial infarction.
43. Mobitz II second-degree AV block occurs almost as frequently with acute myocardial infarction as does the Mobitz I variety.
44. The dose of lidocaine should be reduced in the presence of congestive heart failure.
45. For a malpractice claim to be successful the plaintiff must only establish that a patient-physician relationship existed and that the physician was negligent in the care rendered to the patient.
46. The dose of atropine for a 15 kg infant is 0.075 mg IV.
47. Third-degree AV block that occurs at the level of the AV node (i.e., with an escape rhythm that has a narrow QRS complex) is usually transient and associated with a good prognosis.
48. The esophageal obturator airway is inserted with the patient's head in the sniffing position.
49. The presence of "warning arrhythmias" reliably predicts those patients most likely to develop ventricular fibrillation with acute myocardial infarction.
50. A patient initially has ventricular tachycardia. He is unresponsive, has only a weak pulse, and no blood pressure is obtainable. Lidocaine is the treatment of choice.

ANSWERS AND REFERENCES

The answers given in this section include the page in this book where a discussion or an explanation can be found. Each answer also has a reference in which additional information on the particular question can be obtained. The references used are the *JAMA Supplement* and the American Heart Association's *Textbook of Advanced Cardiac Life Support* (1981).

1. C (p. 3); JAMA, p. 491
2. A, B, C, D, E (p. 7); AHA, p. II-6
3. D; JAMA, p. 461
4. C (p. 13); JAMA, p. 467
5. A, B, C, E (pp. 9, 32); AHA, p. VI-12
6. E (p. 149); AHA, pp. II-6 to II-8
7. E (p. 127); AHA, p. III-2
8. A, C (pp. 28, 175); AHA, p. III-3
9. A (p. 13); JAMA, pp. 467-469
10. B; JAMA, p. 476
11. B (p. 149); AHA, p. II-4
12. B (p. 15); AHA, p. II-5
13. A, B, D (pp. 16, 27); AHA, pp. VIII-2 and VIII-3
14. B (pp. 16, 26); AHA, p. VIII-4
15. A, B, D, E (pp. 30, 46); AHA, pp. VIII-7 and VIII-8
16. B, C, D, E (p. 31); AHA, pp. VIII-8 and VIII-9
17. A, D (pp. 18, 35); AHA, p. IX-3
18. C (p. 127); AHA, pp. X-2 and X-3
19. D; AHA, pp. XII-8 to XII-11
20. A; JAMA, p. 463-465

21. A, B, D; JAMA, p. 476
22. C (p. 38); AHA, p. VII-6
23. A, C; AHA, p. IV-3
24. B; AHA, p. II-1
25. B, C, D, E (pp. 32, 96); AHA, p. VI-23
26. A, D, E (pp. 81-83, 151-152); AHA, pp. VI-13 and VI-14
27. A, D (p. 64); AHA, p. VI-27
28. A, B, C, E (p. 6); AHA, pp. VI-20 and VI-21
29. B, C, E (p. 101); AHA, p. VI-27
30. A, C, E; AHA, p. XII-9
31. False; AHA, p. IV-4
32. True; AHA, pp. IV-4 and IV-5
33. False; AHA, p. III-7
34. True; AHA, p. IV-6
35. True; AHA, p. XII-5
36. True (p. 38); AHA, p. XVII-2
37. False (pp. 17, 32); AHA, p. VIII-10
38. False (pp. 34-35); AHA, p. III-2
39. True (p. 49); AHA, p. III-1
40. False; AHA, p. III-8
41. False; AHA, p. III-7
42. False (p. 163); AHA, p. III-5
43. False (p. 96); AHA, p. III-4
44. True (pp. 30, 43); AHA, pp. VIII-6 and VIII-8
45. False; AHA, pp. XVIII-1 and XVIII-2
46. False (p. 37); AHA, p. XVII-11
47. True (p. 101); AHA, p. VI-25
48. False; AHA, p. IV-2
49. False (pp. 48-49); AHA, p. III-2
50. False (p. 6); AHA, pp. VI-20 and VI-21

DYSRHYTHMIA RECOGNITION QUIZ

1

Lead V$_1$

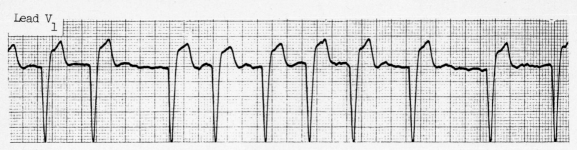

2

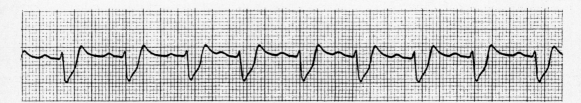

3

Lead II

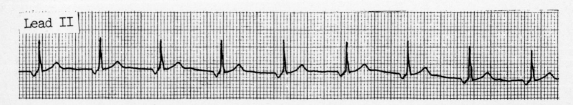

4

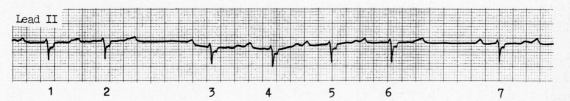

5

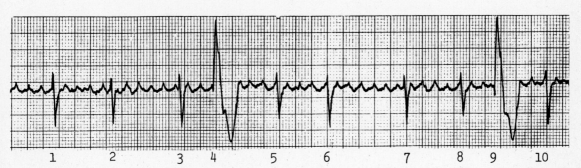

6

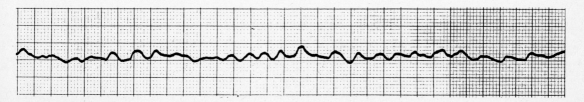

7

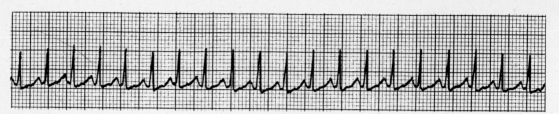

8

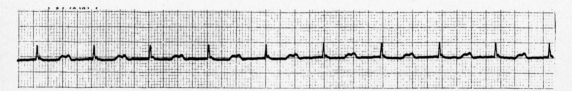

9

Lead V₁

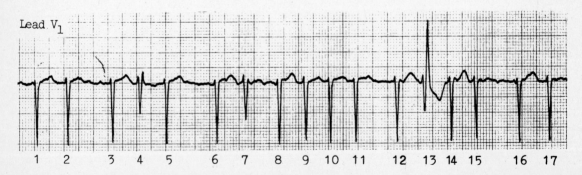

10

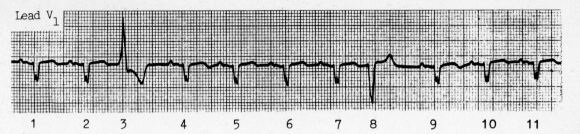

11

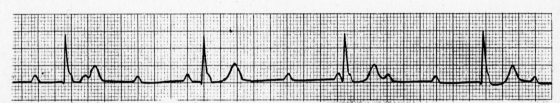

12

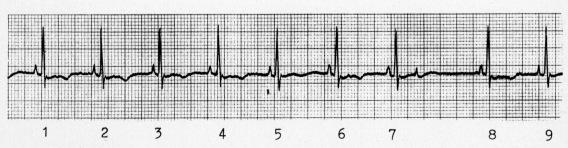

13

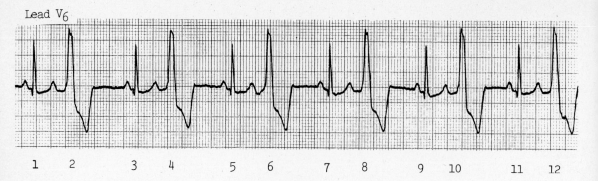

Lead V_6

1 2 3 4 5 6 7 8 9 10 11 12

14

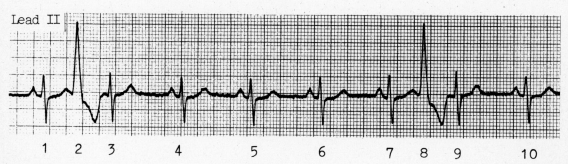

Lead II

1 2 3 4 5 6 7 8 9 10

15

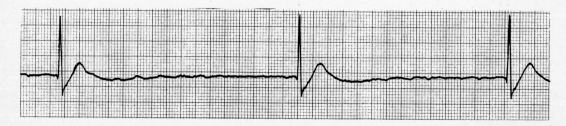

16

Lead MCL₁

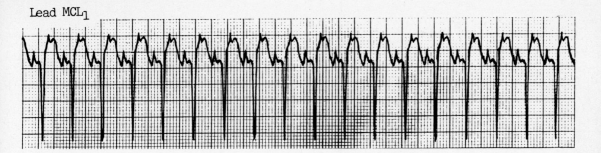

17

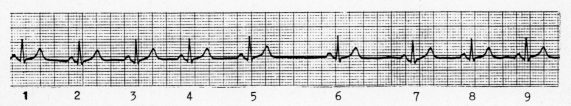

18

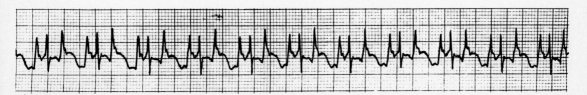

19

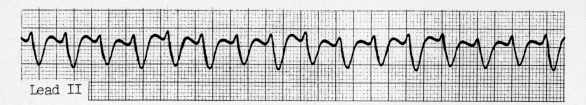

Lead II

20

Lead MCL$_6$

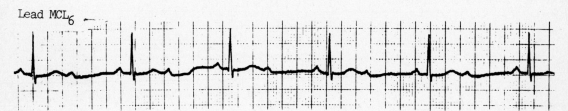

21

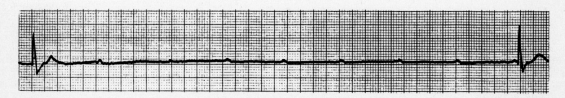

22

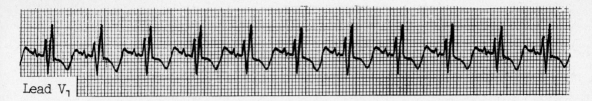

Lead V₁

23

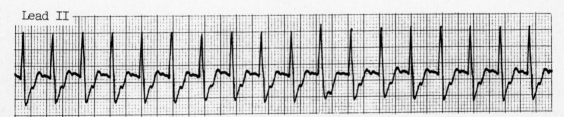

Lead II

24

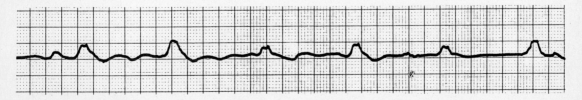

25

Lead MCL₁

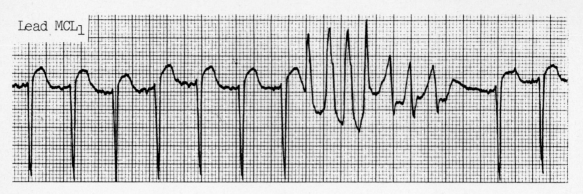

26

Lead V₁

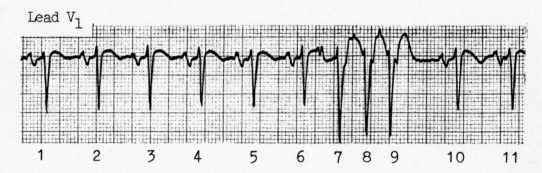

27

Lead MCL₁

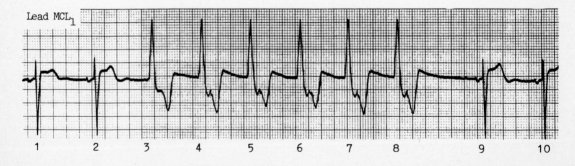

28

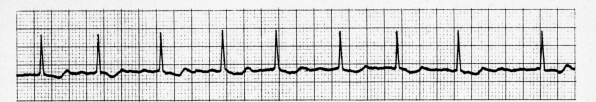

29

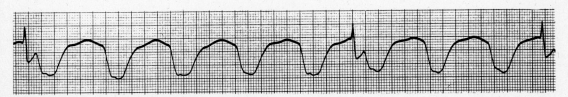

30

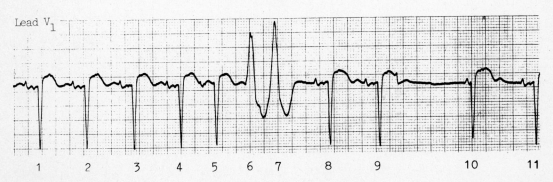

31

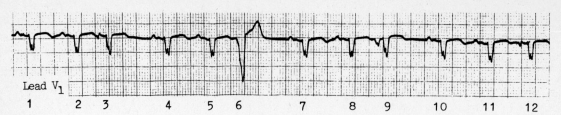

Lead V$_1$
1   2   3   4   5   6   7   8   9   10   11   12

32

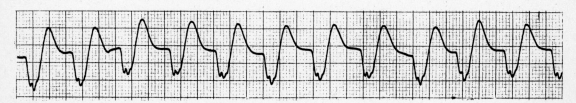

33

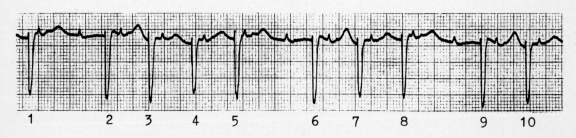

1   2   3   4   5   6   7   8   9   10

34

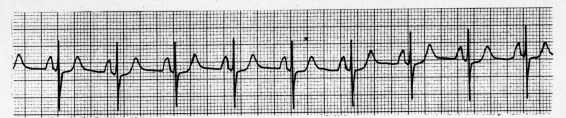

35

Lead MCL$_6$

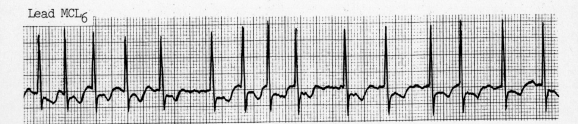

36

Lead II

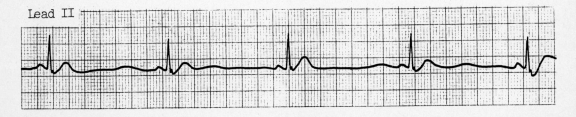

37

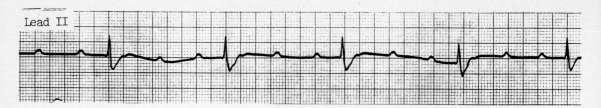

Lead II

38

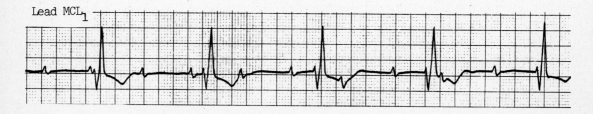

Lead MCL$_1$

39

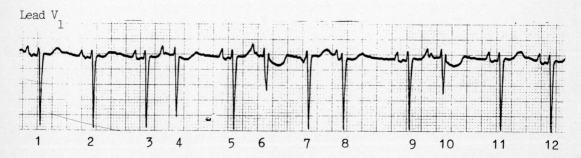

Lead V$_1$

40

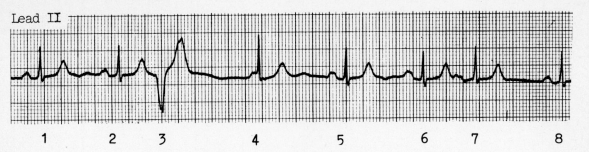

Lead II

1 2 3 4 5 6 7 8

41

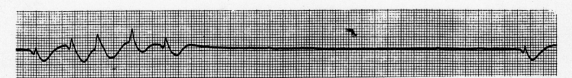

42

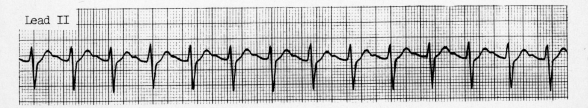

Lead II

43

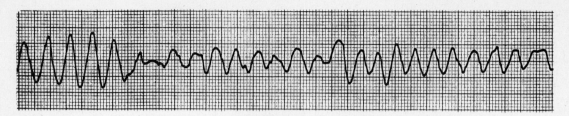

44

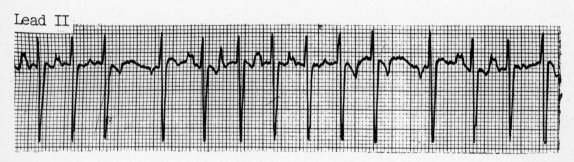

45

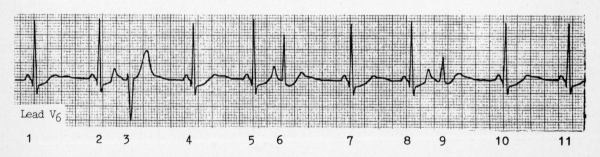

46

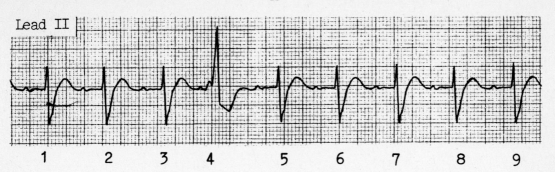

47

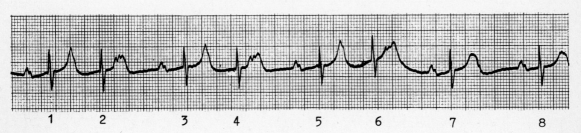

48

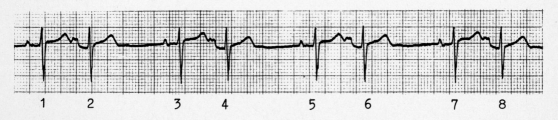

49

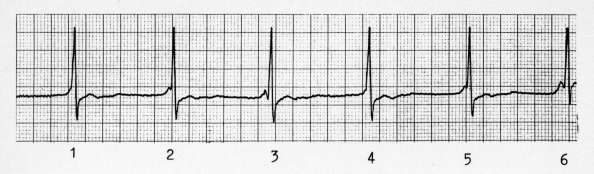

50

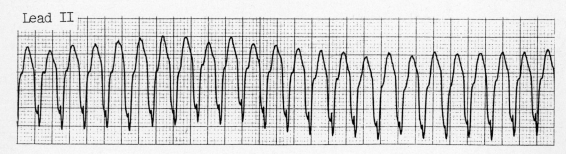

ANSWERS

1. Rhythm—irregularly irregular
   P waves—none
   QRS complex—wide (0.12 second)
   Impression: Atrial fibrillation with a controlled ventricular response.
   Comment: Although many undulations are seen along the baseline, no consistent atrial activity is present. The QRS prolongation is caused by a preexisting left bundle branch block (LBBB).

2. Rhythm—regular
   Rate—85 beats/min
   PR interval—prolonged (0.22 second)
   QRS complex—very wide (0.19 second)
   Impression: Sinus rhythm with first-degree atrioventricular (AV) block.
   Comment: Despite the marked widening of the QRS complex, well-defined P waves precede each beat, identifying the rhythm as sinus.

3. Rhythm—regular
   Rate—80 beats/min
   P waves—inverted; precede the QRS complex with a short PR interval
   QRS complex—normal (≤ 0.10 second)
   Impression: Junctional rhythm.
   Comment: With junctional rhythm, P waves may precede the QRS complex as shown here, follow the QRS complex, or be hidden by their simultaneous occurrence with the QRS complex. Because of the retrograde activation of the atria from the junctional focus, P waves will be inverted in lead II. A low atrial rhythm may also manifest negative P waves in lead II, but the PR interval is usually longer than is shown here.

   The heart rate in this tracing is somewhat faster than one characteristically sees with a junctional rhythm. If the patient was on digitalis, toxicity should be suspected. One cannot be absolutely sure from this rhythm strip alone that the negative deflection is really a P wave and not the initial portion of the QRS complex. If this were the case, the QRS complex would then be widened, and the rhythm would be an accelerated idioventricular rhythm.

4. Rhythm—irregular
   Atrial rate—regular at 70 beats/min
   PR interval—gradually lengthens until a beat is dropped
   QRS complex—borderline prolongation (0.11 second)
   Impression: Second-degree AV block, Mobitz I (Wenckebach).
   Comment: Although the PR interval may not at first appear to be lengthening from beats 3 to 6, comparison of the PR interval of the beat immediately before the pause (beat 6) with the PR interval of the beat that ter-

minates the pause (beat 7) confirms the Wenckebach pattern. The borderline QRS prolongation and configuration in this standard lead II is the result of a left anterior hemiblock.

5. Rhythm—irregular
   Atrial rate—sawtooth flutter waves at 360/min
   QRS complex—normal duration
   Impression: Atrial flutter with a variable ventricular response. Unifocal PVCs (beats 4 and 9).
   Comment: The atrial rate in this example is somewhat faster than one usually sees with atrial flutter.

6. Rhythm—no organized electrical activity.
   Impression: Ventricular fibrillation (fine).

7. Rhythm—regular
   Rate—210 beats/min
   P waves—impossible to determine if the positive deflection preceding each QRS complex
   is a P wave, a T wave, or both
   QRS complex—normal duration
   Impression: Paroxysmal supraventricular tachycardia (PSVT).
   Comment: Although the differential includes paroxysmal atrial tachycardia (PAT), paroxysmal junctional tachycardia (PJT), sinus tachycardia, and atrial flutter, the latter two possibilities are much less likely. Sinus tachycardia rarely goes above 160 beats/min in an adult. The atrial rate in flutter is most often around 300 beats/min (range 250 to 350). A rate of 210 beats/min would be slower than expected if there were 1:1 AV conduction and too fast if there were 2:1 AV conduction.

8. Rhythm—regular
   Rate—75 beats/min
   PR interval—markedly prolonged (0.39 second)
   QRS complex—normal duration
   Impression: Sinus rhythm with first-degree AV block.
   Comment: Although one might interpret this strip as a junctional rhythm, the notch in the T wave is most likely the result of a P wave with a markedly prolonged PR interval.

9. Rhythm—irregularly irregular
   P waves—none
   QRS complex—normal duration
   Impression: Atrial fibrillation with a controlled ventricular response. Beats 4, 7, and 13 are all conducted with aberrancy.
   Comment: Factors favoring aberrancy are a similar initial deflection in the anomalous beats to the normally conducted beats, a typical right bundle branch block (RBBB) pattern (rSR') for beat 13 and an incomplete RBBB pattern for beats 4 and 7 in this right-sided lead, and only minimal prolongation of the QRS complex of these anomalous beats.

10. Rhythm—regular except for beats 3 and 8
    Rate—70 beats/min

PR interval—normal (i.e., between 0.12 and 0.20 second)

QRS complex—normal

Impression: Sinus rhythm. Beats 3 and 8 are premature ventricular contractions (PVCs) from two different foci (multifocal PVCs).

Comment: Beat 3 is clearly a PVC. Although the configuration of beat 8 resembles that of the normally conducted beats, the QRS complex is deeper, the T wave is different, there is no premature P wave, and beat 8 is contained within a full compensatory pause. Therefore beat 8 is most likely a PVC.

11. Atrial rate and rhythm—regular at 100 beats/min
   Ventricular rate and rhythm—regular at 37 beats/min
   PR interval—variable (P waves march through the QRS complex)
   QRS complex—wide (0.12 second)
   Impression: Third-degree (complete) AV block.

12. Rhythm—regular except for the pause between beats 7 and 8
   Rate—80 beats/min
   PR interval—normal
   QRS complex—normal duration
   Impression: Sinus rhythm with a blocked premature atrial contraction (PAC).
   Comment: The most common reason for a pause is a blocked PAC, in this case identified as the notch deforming the T wave that follows beat 7.

13. Rhythm—bigeminy
   PR interval—normal
   QRS complex—normal duration
   Impression: Ventricular bigeminy.
   Comment: Beats 1, 3, 5, 7, 9, and 11 are sinus conducted. The question is posed as to whether beats 2, 4, 6, 8, 10, and 12 are PVCs or PACs that are aberrantly conducted. Factors favoring ventricular ectopy are that these beats are wide and bizarre in configuration with an oppositely directed initial QRS deflection (the sinus conducted beats demonstrate a small negative initial deflection). Finally, no definite premature P waves are evident in front of beats 2, 4, 6, 8, 10, and 12.

   The difficulty arises because one never sees two normally conducted beats in a row. As a result, it is impossible to determine the normal R-R interval. Without knowing what the normal R-R interval should be, one cannot determine if a full compensatory pause exists. In addition, since two normally conducted beats never occur in a row, one cannot be sure what the normal T wave is supposed to look like. This makes it impossible to ascertain if the slightly peaked configuration of the T waves following the odd-numbered beats might be caused by hidden atrial activity. For lack of strong evidence proving aberrancy, one must assume that the even-numbered beats are PVCs.

14. Rhythm—regular except for beats 2 and 8
   Rate—70 beats/min
   PR interval—normal
   QRS complex—normal duration
   Impression: Sinus rhythm with two interpolated PVCs.
   Comment: Beats 2 and 8 are PVCs, since they are wide and bizarre and are not preceded by a premature P wave. They are somewhat unusual in being sandwiched between two normally occurring QRS complexes without producing any postectopic pause (i.e., they are interpolated).

15. Rhythm—slightly irregular
   Rate—about 20 beats/min
   P waves—none
   QRS complex—probably wide, although one cannot be certain where the QRS complex ends and the ST segment begins
   Impression: Slow idioventricular rhythm.

16. Rhythm—regular
   Atrial rate—310 beats/min
   Ventricular rate—155 beats/min
   QRS complex—normal duration
   Impression: Atrial flutter with 2:1 AV conduction.
   Comment: One should strongly consider the diagnosis of atrial flutter with 2:1 AV conduction when confronted with an SVT that has a ventricular response of between 140 and 160 beats/min. In this tracing regularly occurring pointed flutter waves are seen preceding each QRS complex and notching the T wave. Maneuvers to increase vagal tone would be helpful in confirming the diagnosis by slowing down the ventricular response and bringing out the sawtooth configuration of the flutter waves.

   PAT with 2:1 block can usually be differentiated from atrial flutter with 2:1 AV conduction by the slower atrial rate of the former (the atrial rate in PAT is most often between 150 and 250 beats/min) and its isoelectric baseline. At times, however, it is extremely difficult to make this distinction.

17. Rhythm—irregular
   P waves—precede each QRS complex with a constant PR interval
   QRS complex—normal duration
   Impression: Sinus arrhythmia.
   Comment: Sinus arrhythmia is a common normal variant in a pediatric population. In the elderly it may be a manifestation of sick sinus syndrome.

18. Rhythm—irregular
   Rate—up to 400 beats/min
   Impression: Artifact.
   Comment: No organized cardiac rhythm occurs at as rapid a rate as is shown here. Thus this tracing must represent artifact.

19. Rhythm—regular
    Rate—155 beats/min
    P waves—none evident
    QRS complex—wide (0.18 second)
    Impression: Ventricular tachycardia.
    Comment: Although this rhythm could possibly represent SVT with either aberrant conduction or preexisting bundle branch block, ventricular tachycardia must be assumed until proven otherwise.
20. Rhythm—regular
    Atrial rate—90 beats/min
    Ventricular rate—45 beats/min
    QRS complex—normal duration
    Impression: Second-degree AV block with 2:1 AV conduction, either Mobitz I or II.
    Comment: One cannot absolutely differentiate between Mobitz I and II second-degree AV block in the presence of 2:1 AV conduction. The normal QRS duration, however, strongly favors this to be Mobitz I.
21. Rhythm—unable to determine regularity because of the extremely slow ventricular rate
    Atrial rate—varies slightly between 55 and 65 beats/min
    QRS complex—wide (0.12 second)
    Impression: Complete AV block with a long period of ventricular standstill.
22. Rhythm—regular
    Rate—98 beats/min
    PR interval—normal
    QRS complex—prolonged (0.12 second)
    Impression: Sinus rhythm.
    Comment: Although the QRS complex is widened, each beat is preceded by a P wave with a constant PR interval. The rSR' configuration of the QRS complex is the result of a preexisting RBBB. One cannot rule out the possibility that the RBBB is rate related.
23. Rhythm—regular
    Rate—155 beats/min
    P waves—no well-defined P waves are seen, although notching of the baseline may represent atrial activity, possibly flutter
    QRS complex—probably of normal duration although one cannot be certain of where the QRS complex ends and the ST segment begins
    Impression: Regular tachydysrhythmia at 150 beats/min.
    Comment: This is a difficult tracing. The most pressing question is whether the rhythm is supraventricular or ventricular tachycardia. Assuming that the patient is hemodynamically stable, obtaining a 12-lead ECG might be helpful in resolving this issue. If the QRS complex were clearly of normal duration in most leads, the differential would be narrowed down to that of a supraventricular tachycardia (PAT, PJT, sinus tachycardia, or

atrial flutter). On the other hand, if the QRS complex appeared consistently wide in a 12-lead ECG, one would again be faced with the diagnostic dilemma posed previously by tracing 19 of differentiating between ventricular tachycardia and SVT with either aberrant conduction or preexisting bundle branch block.

24. Rhythm—irregular
    P waves—none
    QRS complex—very wide (up to 0.30 second)
    Impression: Agonal rhythm.
    Comment: Although this tracing superficially resembles an idioventricular rhythm, the QRS complexes are extremely wide and formless, suggesting a preterminal state. This is an agonal rhythm.
25. Rhythm—initially regular; interrupted by a run of anomalous beats
    PR interval—normal   } for the first
    QRS complex—normal duration } seven beats
    Impression: Sinus rhythm interrupted by a run of ventricular tachycardia.
    Comment: The QRS morphology varies slightly during the run of anomalous beats. Following a postectopic pause, sinus rhythm resumes.
26. Rhythm—initially regular; interrupted by three anomalous beats (7 to 9)
    PR interval—normal
    QRS interval—normal duration
    Impression: Sinus rhythm interrupted by three aberrantly conducted beats.
    Comment: Beats 7 to 9 are aberrantly conducted rather than being ventricular ectopic beats. They are not markedly widened, they have a similar initial deflection to the normally conducted beats, and a premature P wave that deforms the T wave of beat 6 initiates the sequence. It is difficult to be certain if the notch in the T wave of beats 7 and 8 represents antegrade or retrograde atrial activity.

    As opposed to the more common (and more easily recognized) RBBB pattern of aberration, the anomalous beats in this tracing represent an LBBB pattern of abberration.
27. Rhythm—irregular
    Impression: Sinus rhythm interrupted by a run of accelerated idioventricular rhythm (beats 3 to 8).
    Comment: Following two sinus beats the QRS configuration changes with beat 3. This beat is not premature but is rather an escape beat that arises because of the slight slowing of the sinus pacemaker. Retrograde P waves notch the T waves of beats 4 to 8. After a short pause, sinus rhythm resumes with beat 9.

    Beats 3 to 8 are *not* the result of aberration. There would be no reason for these beats to conduct aberrantly, since they occur so long after the refractory period of beat 2.

28. Rhythm—irregularly irregular
 P waves—none
 QRS complex—normal duration
 Impression: Atrial fibrillation with a controlled ventricular response.
29. Rhythm—irregular
 P waves—none
 QRS complex—probably of normal duration
 Impression: CPR with underlying agonal rhythm.
 Comment: Apart from an occasional agonal complex, one is struck by the regular broad-based negative deflections in the baseline. These occur at a freqency of about 60/min (1/sec) and reflect ongoing CPR.
30. Rhythm—initially regular; interrupted by an early beat (5), two bizarre-looking complexes (beats 6 and 7), and a pause (between beats 9 and 10)
 PR interval—normal
 QRS complex—normal duration
 Impression and Comment: The first four beats are sinus. Beat 5 is a PAC and is followed by two PVCs (beats 6 and 7). The pause after beat 9 is the result of a blocked PAC that deforms the terminal portion of the T wave of this beat. Finally, the PR interval of beat 10 is too short to conduct, suggesting that this QRS complex is a junctional escape beat.
31. Rhythm—irregular
 PR interval—slightly prolonged (0.21 second)
 QRS complex—normal duration
 Impression: Sinus rhythm with first-degree AV block. PACs and a PVC.
 Comment: Beats 3, 9, and 12 are clearly PACs. They occur early and are preceded by P waves yet manifest a QRS configuration identical to that of the normally conducted beats.

Beat 6 is a PVC. It is wider, is more bizarre in shape, and has an oppositely directed initial deflection to that of the normally conducted beats (6 demonstrates a QS morphology that differs from the rS configuration of the normally conducted beats).

There is a full compensatory pause between beats 8 to 10 despite the fact that beat 9 is *not* a PVC. This is a coincidental occurrence that underscores why one should not rely heavily on the finding of a compensatory pause in the differentiation of PVCs from aberrancy.

32. Rhythm—fairly regular
 P waves—appear to notch the QRS complex
 Ventricular rate—about 100 beats/min
 QRS complex—wide (0.17 second)
 Impression: Ventricular tachycardia.
 Comment: The finding of P waves that notch each QRS complex does not assist in the differential diagnosis of this wide complex tachydysrhythmia. One must assume the rhythm to be ventricular tachycardia until proven otherwise.
33. Rhythm—irregular
 Atrial rate—regular at 115/min
 QRS complex—normal duration
 Impression: Second-degree AV block Mobitz I.
 Comment: Although one may be tempted to attribute the pauses that follow beats 1, 5, and 8 to blocked PACs, the P waves that notch the T waves of these beats are *not* premature. The following figure (51) indicates that each QRS complex is in fact preceded by a P wave with a progressively lengthening PR interval until a beat is dropped.

Two reasons the Wenckebach phenomenon is harder to recognize in this tracing are that the atrial rate is faster than usual and the PR interval is markedly prolonged.

51

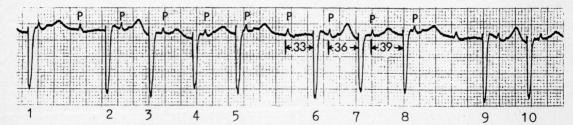

34. Rhythm—regular
    Rate—85 beats/min
    PR interval—normal
    QRS complex—normal duration
    Impression: Sinus rhythm.
    Comment: The shape of the T wave resembles that of the P wave, suggesting that 2:1 AV conduction might exist. However, use of calipers to measure the P-T interval reveals that it differs from the T-P interval. Thus this is simply a sinus rhythm.

35. Rhythm—irregularly irregular
    P waves—none
    QRS complex—normal duration
    Impression: Atrial fibrillation with a moderately rapid ventricular response.

36. Rhythm—regular
    Rate—40 beats/min
    PR interval—normal
    QRS complex—normal duration.
    Impression: Sinus bradycardia.

37. Atrial rate and rhythm—114 beats/min and regular
    Ventricular rate and rhythm—38 beats/min and regular
    QRS complex—wide (0.13 second)
    Impression: High-grade second-degree AV block, Mobitz II.
    Comment: Although severe impairment of AV conduction is present, each QRS complex that does occur is preceded by a P wave with a constant PR interval. Thus the degree of AV block cannot be complete.

38. Atrial rate and rhythm—88 beats/min
    Ventricular rate and rhythm—40 beats/min
    QRS complex—wide (0.16 second)
    Impression: Third-degree (complete) AV block.
    Comment: As opposed to tracing 37, the PR interval in this tracing continuously varies (the P wave marches through the QRS complex). This is complete AV block.

39. Rhythm—irregular
    PR interval—normal
    QRS complex—normal duration
    Impression: Sinus rhythm with PACs, most of which conduct with aberrancy.
    Comment: The first three beats demonstrate an underlying sinus rhythm at 80 beats/min. Beats 4, 6, 8, and 10 are all PACs. The premature P waves of beats 6 and 10 occur earlier during the relative refractory period than the P wave of beat 8 and consequently are conducted with a greater degree of aberrancy.

40. Rhythm—irregular
    PR interval—normal
    QRS complex—normal duration
    Impression and Comment: The first two beats are sinus. Beat 3 is a PVC. It is wide, is bizarre in shape, and demonstrates a QRS configuration that is oppositely directed to the normally conducted beats.

    The P wave preceding beat 4 occurs on time but with a PR interval that is too short to conduct. Although beat 4 differs slighly in configuration from the other beats, it has a similar initial deflection, it has a similar T wave, and it is not really widened. It is a junctional escape beat that occurred before the P wave preceding it could be conducted to the ventricles. Beat 7 is a PAC.

41. Rhythm—irregular
    P waves—none
    QRS complex—wide (0.16 second)
    Impression: Agonal rhythm with a long period of asystole.

42. Rhythm—regular
    Rate—112 beats/min
    PR interval—normal (0.17 second)
    QRS complex—borderline prolongation (0.11 second)
    Impression: Sinus tachycardia.
    Comment: Although not obvious, P waves follow each T wave (arrows in following illustration [52]).

43. Rhythm—irregular
    Impression: Ventricular flutter rapidly degenerating to coarse ventricular fibrillation.

52

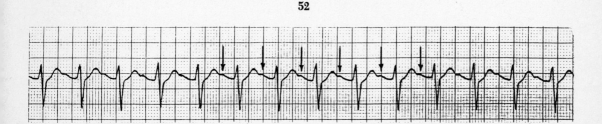

44. Rhythm—irregularly irregular
 P waves—continuously varying in morphology
 QRS complex—normal duration
 Impression: Multifocal atrial tachycardia (chaotic atrial mechanism).
 Comment: The irregular irregularity of the rhythm at first suggests atrial fibrillation. However, unlike atrial fibrillation, definite P waves are present, albeit with a continuously changing morphology and varying PR interval.

45. Rhythm—trigeminy
 PR interval—normal
 QRS complex—normal duration
 Impression: Atrial trigeminy with aberrant conduction.
 Comment: Beats 3, 6, and 9 are not PVCs because they are not widened and are all clearly preceded by a premature P wave that deforms the T wave of beats 2, 5, and 8. Beats 3 and 9 are conducted with a greater degree of aberrancy than beat 6, since their premature P waves occur earlier during the relative refractory period.

There is an initial negative deflection (q wave) to the normally conducted beats. This is one example of aberrancy in which the initial deflection of the aberrantly conducted QRS complex differs from that of the normally conducted beats.

46. Rhythm—regular except for beat 4
 Rate—95 beats/min
 PR interval—slightly prolonged (0.21 second)
 QRS complex—wide (0.12 second)
 Impression: Sinus rhythm with first-degree AV block and a PVC.
 Comment: The P wave preceding beat 4 occurs precisely on time, but it has a PR interval that is too short to conduct (see the following illustration [53]). Thus beat 4 must arise from either the AV node or the ventricles. Since the morphology of this beat greatly differs from that of the normally conducted beats, it must be a PVC.

53

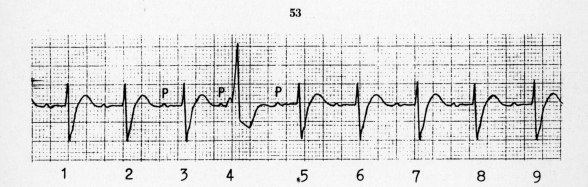

47. Rhythm—regularly irregular (group beating)
Atrial rate—regular at 98 beats/min (see the following illustration [54])
QRS complex—normal duration
Impression: Second-degree AV block Mobitz I.
Comment: The pattern of group beating seen here should immediately raise one's suspicion for a Wenckebach type of conduction disturbance. The following illustration demonstrates the regularity of atrial activity and the gradually lengthening PR interval until a beat is dropped.

48. Rhythm—regularly irregular (group beating)
Atrial rate—irregular
QRS complex—normal duration
Impression: Atrial bigeminy.
Comment: As in tracing 47, the phenomenon of group beating should suggest the possibility of a Wenckebach type of conduction disturbance. However, unlike the previous example, the atrial activity in this tracing is not regular. The P waves that precede beats 2, 4, 6, and 8 are all premature and differ in morphology from the P waves of the odd-numbered beats. Thus they represent PACs rather than a type of AV block.

49. Rhythm—almost regular
Atrial and ventricular rates—almost equal at about 53 beats/min

54

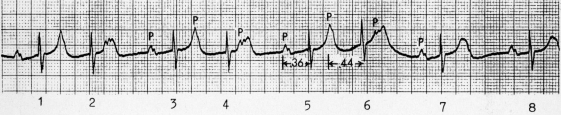

P waves—occur before each QRS complex with a slightly varying PR interval that is too short to conduct
QRS complex—normal duration
Impression: Isorhythmic AV dissociation.
Comment: AV dissociation is present, since the PR interval varies and there is no consistent relation between atrial and ventricular activity (see the following illustration [55]). Because of the close proximity of atrial and junctional rates, this rhythm is termed *isorhythmic AV dissociation*.

It is impossible to determine the degree of AV block present (if any) from this tracing alone, since none of the P waves are given an adequate opportunity to conduct (i.e., the PR intervals are too short to allow normal AV conduction).

50. Rhythm—regular
Rate—230 beats/min
P waves—none
QRS complex—wide (0.14 second)
Impression: Ventricular tachycardia.
Comment: As with tracing 19, the differential diagnosis of a regular, wide complex tachydysrhythmia includes ventricular tachycardia and SVT with either aberrant conduction or a preexisting bundle branch block. Ventricular tachycardia must be assumed until proven otherwise.

55

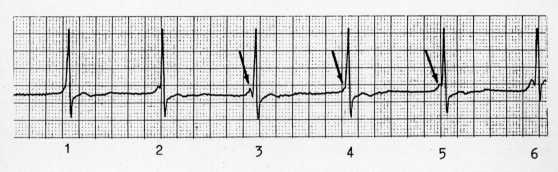

1   2   3   4   5   6

ADVANCED LIFE SUPPORT POCKET GUIDE

The algorithms and basic drugs used in cardiopulmonary resuscitation are consolidated in the following boxes. These may be cut on the lines and laminated for use as a pocket reference.

Drugs used in Cardiac Arrest

Epinephrine (1 ampule = 10 ml = 1 mg)—0.5-1.0 mg (5-10 ml of 1:10,000 solution) by IV or ET tube

Sodium Bicarbonate (1 ampule = 50 mEq)—1 mEq/kg initially; ½ dose every 10 min; *appropriate* sodium bicarbonate depends on ABGs

Atropine—0.5-1.0 mg IV (or by ET tube) every 5 min up to 2 mg

Calcium chloride (1 ampule = 1000 mg = 10 ml)—500 mg IV (5 ml of 10% solution); may repeat once in 10 min

Lidocaine—1 mg/kg (50-100 mg) initial IV bolus; may repeat 50-75 mg boluses every 5-10 min 2 times

Procainamide—100 mg increments IV slowly over 5 min up to 1 g (watch QRS widening, hypotension), or infuse 500-1000 mg over 30 min

Bretylium (1 ampule = 500 mg)—5-10 mg/kg (about 500 mg) IV bolus; may repeat every 15-30 min up to 30 mg/kg; drug takes up to 15 min to work; apply countershock after bolus

For VT dilute 500 mg bretylium in 50 ml D_5W, and infuse over 10 min

Verapamil—5-10 mg (0.75-0.150 mg/kg) IV over 1-4 min period; may repeat once in 30 min

IV INFUSION RATES

Lidocaine—
Bretylium } 1 g in 250 ml D_5W (= 2 g in 500 ml); begin drip at 15-30 drops/min (= 1-2 mg/min)
Procainamide

Isoproterenol—
Epinephrine } 1 mg in 250 ml D_5W; begin drip at 15-30 drops/min (= 1-2 μg/min)

Dopamine— 200 mg (= 1 ampule) in 250 ml D_5W; begin drip at 30 drops/min (= 5 μg/kg/min for an 80 kg patient)

Sodium nitroprusside—
nitroglycerin } 50 mg in 250 ml D_5W (= 200 μg/ml); begin drip at 3 drops/min (= 10 μg/min); may increase infusion rate by 3 drops/min (10μg/min) every 5 min

Ventricular Fibrillation (V FIB)

Countershock at 200 J 2 times
CPR
Epinephrine
Sodium bicarbonate
Countershock at 360 J
Bretylium (500 mg IV)
CPR; then reshock at 360 J
Epinephrine
Sodium bicarbonate
Bretylium (500-1000 mg IV)
CPR; then reshock at 360 J
Lidocaine bolus and infusion (or bretylium
  infusion) as soon as patient converts to sta-
  ble rhythm

Precordial thump—only indicated when onset of VT or V FIB is monitored

Ventricular Tachycardia (VT)

No pulse—treat as V FIB
Hypotensive—cardioversion at 200 J
Alert, good BP—Lidocaine (may repeat)
  Procainamide
  Bretylium
  Cardioversion at 50-
  200 J

SVT/Rapid Atrial Fibrillation

Verapamil (carotid massage for SVT)
Digoxin
Propranolol
Cardioversion

Asystole

CPR
Epinephrine
Sodium bicarbonate
Atropine (1 mg 2 times)
Repeat epinephrine
Calcium chloride
Pacemaker insertion

Bradydysrhythmias
(AV block; slow idioventricular rhythm)

Atropine
Isoproterenol (or epinephrine or dopamine)
Pacemaker insertion

Electromechanical Dissociation (EMD)

CPR
Epinephrine
Sodium bicarbonate
Look for underlying cause:
  right mainstem bronchus intubation
  tension pneumothorax
  cardiac tamponade
  acidosis, $\uparrow K^+$, $\downarrow K^+$
  pulmonary embolus
  ruptured aortic aneurysm
  cardiogenic shock
  hypovolemic shock

Consider fluid challenge and/or treatment of other underlying cause
Repeat epinephrine
Calcium chloride

Index